Lidiana Macêdo Holanda
Ana Caroline de Sousa
Gustavo Cardoso da Silva Neves

Microbiological Biotechnology in Aesthetic Microneedling

Lidiana Macêdo Holanda
Ana Caroline de Sousa
Gustavo Cardoso da Silva Neves

Microbiological Biotechnology in Aesthetic Microneedling

Aesthetic Health

ScienciaScripts

Imprint
Any brand names and product names mentioned in this book are subject to trademark, brand or patent protection and are trademarks or registered trademarks of their respective holders. The use of brand names, product names, common names, trade names, product descriptions etc. even without a particular marking in this work is in no way to be construed to mean that such names may be regarded as unrestricted in respect of trademark and brand protection legislation and could thus be used by anyone.

Cover image: www.ingimage.com

This book is a translation from the original published under ISBN 978-613-9-72656-1.

Publisher:
Sciencia Scripts
is a trademark of
Dodo Books Indian Ocean Ltd. and OmniScriptum S.R.L publishing group

120 High Road, East Finchley, London, N2 9ED, United Kingdom
Str. Armeneasca 28/1, office 1, Chisinau MD-2012, Republic of Moldova, Europe
Printed at: see last page
ISBN: 978-620-7-90212-5

SUMMARY

CHAPTER 1	2
CHAPTER 2	5
CHAPTER 3	8
CHAPTER 4	14
CHAPTER 5	16
CHAPTER 6	20
CHAPTER 7	22
CHAPTER 8	28
CHAPTER 9	33
CHAPTER 10	40
CHAPTER 11	42

CHAPTER 1

Microorganisms and Dermarroler

Scientific studies of microorganisms in terms of their metabolic, physiological and genetic aspects provide support for recognising isolated microorganisms in clinical diagnoses. Macroscopic and microscopic morphologies are the main aspects of microorganisms, but the procedure for identifying the cause of an infection is much broader and more complex, where the patient, signs and symptoms are assessed, as well as the results obtained through physical diagnosis, which presuppose an infection. Although micro-organisms can be identified using various laboratory techniques, the most common way of obtaining results is by isolating micro-organisms in culture using biochemical tests.

Bacteria are the most numerous microorganisms in the environment and in human beings. They are present in many places and can be important for the performance of the body's functions, but they must be in balance. Bacteria are prokaryotic organisms that reproduce by asexual division. They are classified as Gram-positive and Gram-negative. These bacteria can be part of the normal microbiota, but some of these microorganisms can be harmful to human health and can lead to serious pathogens such as **staphylococcus, streptococcus, Escherichia coli** and **Enterobacteriaceae.** Some of these microorganisms, even though they are part of the skin's normal microbiota, are considered to be a type of bacterium responsible for causing widespread bacterial infections that are of concern to human health, as in the case of **staphylococcus, and** skin infections such as topical dermatitis, psoriasis, acne and others have been linked to a disturbance in the skin's normal microbiota and the expansion of infectious microorganisms, such as **Stapylococcus aureu.** These micro-organisms have the capacity to be transmitted by various means, whether through hands or contaminated professional instruments, as in the case of the aesthetic technique of microneedling.

Contamination associated with products must be analysed taking into account the purpose of use, the circumstances of the practices, the frequency and time of product handling. An infection depends on conditions such as the quantity of microorganisms accessible and their degree of pathogenicity. For microbial quality product applications, it is essential to ensure that the microbial load is as low as possible, and that there are no pathogenic microorganisms within legally permitted limits. The prior diagnosis and accelerated identification of microorganisms are essential for the proper control of body infections. There are conventional methods that can take up to 48 hours to identify them, as they multiply at a high rate, and some bacterial strains can present 100 generations in up to 24 hours.

This transmission can occur at the moment when the professional is carrying out a direct method with the patient or through the dissemination of these beings through the environment. For these reasons, it is always important to maintain the hygiene of the equipment used directly and the environment where the procedure is taking place. The recommendations for beauty professionals follow basic biosafety rules such as washing hands, wearing gloves, masks, goggles, aprons, disposing of contaminated material, and care must be taken when there is a risk or not, such as in the presence of blood, secretions and excretions from the skin and mucous membranes.

Health surveillance is responsible for developing activities that can eliminate, reduce or prevent health risks. And to interfere in health problems such as the asepsis, sterilisation and disposal of aesthetic materials and instruments that pose a risk of infection by micro-organisms, contamination resulting from an insignificant volume of blood from small injuries or not to the health professional, so it is up to health surveillance to monitor the circumstances during these activities and determine biosafety standards, preventing the re-use of aesthetic materials and instruments, which can carry infectious agents and cause serious dermatological injuries, therefore an irregular procedure for the health agencies.

The skin is the largest organ that makes up the human body, it covers and delimits the organism, it accounts for 15% of the total weight of the human body and its basic principle is to balance the internal environment, protecting and interacting with the external environment. It is made up of three tissue layers: the upper layer (epidermis), the middle layer (dermis) and the deep layer (subcutaneous cellular tissue).

In recent years there have been major advances in facial rejuvenation techniques, offering professionals more options for improving skin quality. It's common knowledge that everyone wants to have healthy, lush, radiant skin, free of blemishes and scars or any other aesthetic dysfunction. With all this progress, new treatments have emerged that make it possible to have better quality skin free of imperfections. Techniques have been innovated with the aim of disrupting or removing the stratum corneum and thus increasing skin permeability for larger, water-soluble molecules via the transepidermal route. Among these techniques we can mention microneedling, which acts directly on the aesthetics of the skin in the treatment of facial rejuvenation, stretch marks, acne scars and gynoid lipodystrophy. As a skin aesthetics option, this type of procedure can be carried out safely in a dermatologist's clinic by any professional with minimal training.

The micro-needles have a diameter of around 300 gm and a length of between 50 gm and 900 gm, which is enough to make them effective at penetrating and opening small holes only in the layers of the stratum corneum and the viable epidermis of the skin, without damaging the nerve endings located in the dermis. The procedure takes around 15 to 40 minutes depending on the size of the area to be treated. The healing process of the damaged sites in the superficial layers of the skin takes place more quickly than when the procedure is carried out with hypodermic needles, thus avoiding microbial infections. One of the main advantages of using the technique is that the devices can be handled without the help of another professional, and the fact that the technique is painless favours its wide acceptance by patients, especially children.

Also known as percutaneous collagen induction therapy, the Dermaroller is a microneedling technique that emerged in the 1990s in Germany, but only became known worldwide in 2006. In recent years it has become famous as a very simple and effective way of treating scars, especially acne scars, which consists of procedures that have both aesthetic solutions and medical applications. The equipment is based on a plastic roller covered with fine steel or titanium alloy needles, depending on the brand found on the market. The needles can be of various diameters, varying in size from 0.5 to 3 mm and can contain from 190 to 540 parallel needles that are inserted into the epidermis, causing a local inflammatory process and subsequently producing collagen, As recommended by the health authorities, the equipment cannot be reused and is therefore disposable, due to the wide range of risks it can cause through microorganisms that may develop on the equipment. The roller will be slid vertically, horizontally and diagonally about 10 to 15 times in each direction, applying moderate pressure until it injures the skin.

After the injury caused by the needle puncture, cells of the immune system are activated and migrate to the established site, developing cellular metabolism and the synthesis of collagen and elastin by stimulating peripheral blood circulation, consequently repairing and readjusting the supporting fibres, restoring the integrity of the skin.

This process consists of three phases: in the first, injury occurs, where platelets and neutrophils are activated, causing the release of growth factors that influence keratinocytes and fibroblasts, such as transforming growth factors a and b (TGF-a and TGF-b), the growth factor from platelets and protein III, which activates the connective tissue growth factor. In the second phase, known as the healing phase, monocytes replace neutrophils and the process of blood vessel formation from pre-existing vessels takes place, known as angiogenesis, as well as epithelialisation and fibroblast proliferation, followed by the production of type III collagen, elastin, glycosaminoglycans and proteoglycans, and fibroblast growth factor. Around five days after the injury, the fibronectin matrix is fully formed and collagen is deposited just below the basal layer of the epidermis. In the third phase, known as the maturation phase, type III collagen, which is predominant in the first phase of the healing process, is slowly replaced by type I collagen, which is a longer-lasting process, lasting an average of five to seven years.

The restitution of the tissue formed after a lesion in the epithelial tissue begins instantaneously after the loss of the communicative relationship between the adjacent cells, with the release of chemotactic elements, which are mediators that act directly in the inflammatory process, leading to the migration of cells from the vascular and connective tissue.

There are several causes that can lead to complications or undesirable effects in the microneedling process, such as a variation in the choice of equipment, performing the procedure incorrectly, for example: inadequate speed or rhythm for carrying out the technique, overabundant pressure, use of cosmetics or other substances with the potential to induce an allergen, short intervals between sessions, incorrect simultaneous use with other therapeutic means and reuse of needles where it can cause transmission of transmissible diseases or contamination of the patient by some microbial agent. This technique is contraindicated in situations of: warts, herpes or active acne, cancerous lesions, psoriasis, skin disorder and infection, propensity to keloids, pregnant women, diabetics, vitiligo and cushing's syndrome due to excess fat around the face.

CHAPTER 2

Evolution of the Dermarroller

Skin treatment through topical therapy and invasive surgery have specific indications. Ablative procedures aimed at stimulating and remodelling collagen have long been recommended by dermatology. However, nowadays there is a trend towards less invasive procedures, aimed at reducing complications and promoting the patient's rapid return to daily activities. Modalities using lasers, peels and dermabrasion are based on removing the epidermis to trigger cell proliferation through collagen production, with the aim of replacing scarred or aged tissue.

The skin is a formidable natural barrier that was developed to protect the human body. It is made up of three layers, the epidermis (50-150 **pm thick), the dermis** (1-2 mm thick) and the subcutaneous tissue, giving a total skin thickness of approximately 3 mm. The epidermis is the outer skin layer and provides the skin's main barrier. There are five sub-layers of the epidermis including the stratum corneum, stratum lucidum, stratum granulosum, stratum spinosum and stratum basale. The stratum corneum is the skin's main barrier made up of 15-20 stratified layers of corneocytes, surrounded by lipids and enriched in proteins.

It's common knowledge that the search for healthy, lush, radiant skin, free of blemishes and scars or any other aesthetic dysfunction has been increasing in recent years. Some treatments provide better quality skin free of imperfections. Microneedling is a treatment option for various aesthetic skin dysfunctions, such as acne scars, facial rejuvenation, stretch marks and gynoid lipodystrophy.

The use of needles for non-ablative skin treatment was first described by Orentreich and Orentreich in 1995 as subcision surgery, which is the release of depressed scars and wrinkles by needle stimulation. This controlled trauma leads to the formation of tissue to fill the gap created and ligation of the underlying tissue. In 1996, Fernandes used micro-needles organised in a roll, with 3 mm needles, in order to stimulate fibroblasts in the deep reticular layer. However, this needle length proved to be painful, causing persistent bleeding and haematomas on the patient's skin. In 2008 he improved the equipment with 1mm needles, showing similar results in terms of collagen production with the advantage of less downtime, swelling and pain.

Traditionally used as a collagen induction therapy for facial scars and skin rejuvenation, microneedling is currently being extended to transdermal delivery systems for therapeutic drugs and vaccines. Microneedling has been the subject of several clinical trials investigating its effects on atrophic acne scars, skin rejuvenation, burn scars, stretch marks, androgenetic alopecia and melasma.

The treatment is carried out by perforating the stratum corneum, without damaging the epidermis. This process allows the release of growth factors that will encourage the production of collagen and elastin in the papillary dermis. In addition, microneedling is a virtually painless, simple and minimally invasive technique. In this context, it is a good option and its principle is to stimulate collagen production without causing the total de-epithelialisation seen in some ablative techniques.

Microneedling is a technique classified on the basis of multiple parameters including material composition, applications, manufacturing technique and design. The materials used to manufacture the equipment can be based on metal (stainless steel), polymer, glass and silicon, with the manufacturing technique consisting of engraving, injection moulding, micromechanisation, micromoulding and lithography electroforming replication. The design of the equipment can be hollow or solid, the latter with the possibility of being coated or uncoated. The current market is growing with a variety of devices based on needle length, roll size and automation.

Dermarollers are plastic cylinders (2X2 cm) made up of micro-needles. There are a wide variety of brands of these rollers on the market, with variations in the number of needles (192 to 1074), where the length varies from 0.25 to 3 mm and 0.1-0.25 mm in diameter, and they are used in just one application, with the instrument pre-sterilised by gamma irradiation, as the equipment is discarded after use. It is forbidden to reuse or sterilise the Dermaroller, as after use the needles lose their thread and during the autoclaving process they lose their pointed shape and can easily detach from the roller.

It's a simple piece of equipment in which the area to be treated has to be thoroughly cleaned and anaesthetised with topical ointment that should remain on the treatment site for 45 to 1 hour. Once the area to be applied has been prepared, the equipment is rolled 15 to 20 times in horizontal, vertical and oblique directions. The small droplets of blood that form due to the lesions are quick and easy to control. At the end of the technique, which lasts around 15 to 40 minutes depending on the site being treated, the entire area is moistened at the end of the treatment.

There are many micro-organisms that can be transmitted and spread by beauty services, including the skin and mucous membranes with abrasions and wounds. Since microneedling is an aesthetic technique that creates microchannels using a cylindrical roller with microneedles (dermaroller), the recommendations for aesthetic professionals are in line with basic biosafety standards, and care must be taken when there are risks, such as the presence of blood, secretions and excretions from the skin and mucous membranes.

The negative effects or risks arising from microneedling are the reactivation of herpes simplex; impetigo; contact dermatitis allergic to the material used in the needles; exposure to bleeding; equipment with low-quality needles that during the rolling process often results in defects in the tips, causing tissue damage; haemorrhage with hypertrophic scars or post-inflammatory hyperpigmentation. Due to the small skin lesions, there is a potential risk of infection and this should be discussed with the patient beforehand.

Skin infections involve a wide variety of aetiological agents and multiple pathogenic mechanisms. These infections are classified as primary or secondary (depending on whether or not there was an entry point prior to the infection), acute or chronic (depending on the duration of the infection), and can also be mono- or polymicrobial. Infections that have their primary focus in deep structures can manifest as skin rashes. Primary infections occur in patients with no obvious point of entry (e.g. erysipelas). Secondary infections occur as complications of skin lesions (abrasions), surgical trauma or penetrating wounds. These infections can be either monomicrobial, such as wounds infected by staphylococci, or polymicrobial, as in some gangrenous conditions caused by microaerophilic and anaerobic streptococci. Secondary infections can be localised or disseminated, depending on the extent of the underlying diseases, or precipitated by trauma.

The risks of contamination associated with products must be analysed in the light of the need for their use. Microbial transmission is a problem that influences both customer self-confidence and the quality of the product, equipment and so on. It is necessary to ensure that the microbial load is probably lower than legally permitted, as well as the absence of pathogenic microorganisms.

CHAPTER 3

Dermaroller

Micro-needling, known as microneedling, collagen induction therapy or dermaroller, is an invasive and relatively innovative procedure when it comes to aesthetic procedures. It is used through controlled intradermal perforations, by means of fine miniature needles rolling over the skin. This procedure has gained acceptance and popularity among professionals because it is simple to handle, low cost, safe to use correctly and does not necessarily require advanced training, emphasising its promising qualities.

It has a wide range of indications and is commonly used in collagen-inducing treatments for facial scars and skin rejuvenation, including acne and/or acne scars, wrinkles, burns, alopecia, dermal drug use, hyperhidrosis, stretch marks and others.

This method has undergone extensive innovation over the years since it was first used with the initial instrument for microneedling. Since this innovation, it can be combined with other surgical procedures to obtain more satisfactory results. It is preferable to use it on darker skin types, as there is a greater risk of post-inflammatory pigmentation due to techniques that damage the epidermis.

The best and main characteristic of microneedling is that it offers a minimally invasive and painless form of treatment, allowing the best contact between the drug and the applied site, for the main reason that this technology allows microchannels to be created in the skin, so that proteins don't cross the intact skin.

From the moment it becomes a vehicle for active ingredients, it becomes important in the proliferation of skin cells, as well as cell migration, inflammation, angiogenesis, melanogenesis and regulated protein synthesis. In order to have the best biological effect, it needs to be delivered directly and in the most stable form possible, which is why it is of interest because it excludes the first-pass mechanism as well as sustained therapeutic action, overcoming barriers in the stratum corneum.

THE INVESTMENT

The first reports of the use of microneedling began in the 1990s, by Camirand and Doucet, using it on tattoos without pigmentation for the possible treatment of hypertrophic and matic scars. In 1995, Orentreich and Orentreich made more advanced use of it as a method of subcutaneous weakening of scars, using a tri-bevelled hypodermic needle, resulting in the normal course of healing. With the intention of smoothing out post-surgical imperfections, in 2000 the German Liebl proposed a new format for the device. And finally, in 2006, plastic surgeon Fernandes gave the **dermarroller a** new shape, in the form of a drum with multiple thin, protruding needles, with the aim of inducing collagen production.

The evolution of a simple dermarroller, figure 1, over the last decade has seen a variety of changes in shape, along with the demand for the use of this device, with the main changes being in the length of the needles, the size of the drum and the automation. The length of the needles is one of the fundamental factors in this need for change, taking into account the length of the tip in contrast to the diameter, which should be around 13/1 respectively, qualifying good needles. Only the patient's skin type will determine the right **dermarroller.**

As is routine for patients undergoing treatments for acne and other scars, it is usual to use needles with lengths of 1.5 to 2 mm. This ratio changes when indicated to patients undergoing treatments for skin ageing and wrinkles, ranging from around 0.5 to 1 mm, as recommended. Needles of around 0.5 mm cause the least possible pain, which can increase simultaneously as the needles penetrate further, depending on the thickness of the epidermis.

FIGURA 1   Different types of dermarrollers. On the left, dermarroller with a small proportion of drums used in smaller areas, in the middle the device with 540 needles and on the right the standard dermarroller used.

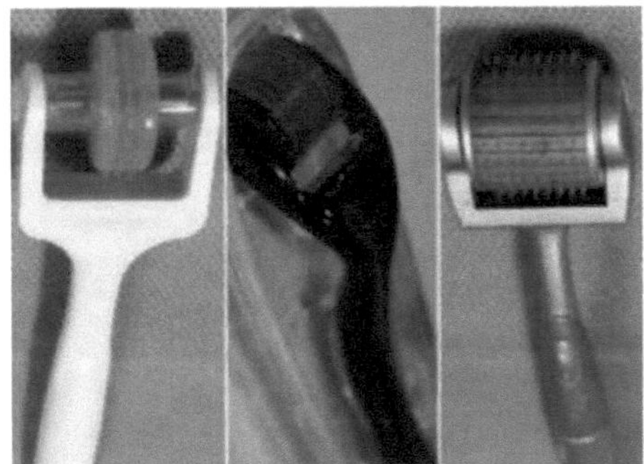

BASIC **DERMARROLLER**

Called the C-8 classified by the Food and Drug Administration, it has a 12 cm long handle, measuring 2x2 cm in width, with a drum-like cylinder shape, with 8 rows and 24 circular matrices, with a total of 192 needles, these needles ranging in length from 0.5 to 3 mm and in diameter from 0.1 to 0.25 mm. Because they are only used once, these needles are synthesised in a unique way, using reactive ions, a corrosion technique on silicon, which can be medium-grade, and stainless steel.

More precisely, this instrument needs to be pre-sterilised by gamma irradiation. As far as the procedure is concerned, rolling with a standard containing 192 needles of 2mm in length and 0.07mm in diameter, with bearings around 15 times, it is possible to obtain a result of around 250 punctures per square metre, depending on the intensity this quantity can vary, each bearing can produce 16 punctures in the stratum corneum per square cm, without damaging the epidermis.

DERMARROLLERS OR DERMA STAMPS

It can be called a home-care **dermarroller**, and has the characteristic of being less than 0.15 mm long, with availability for transdermal delivery of substances such as lipopeptides, as well as other substances that slow down ageing. It can be used twice a week for up to a hundred times. After use, the roller must be cleaned under running water at high temperatures and dried by shaking, although there are peptide-based roller cleaners.

There are a total of 480 needles, 0.2 mm long and 3 mm in diameter, with their barrels strategically separated and placed inside a computer mouse shaped device. It has been designed to ensure ample contact space, making it possible to use it on areas such as the arms, legs and buttocks, and it is effective in treating cellulite on the stomach and thighs.

TYPES C-8HE, CIT-8, MF-8 AND MS-4 LAUNCHED BY THE FDA (FOOD AND DRUG ADMINISTRATION)

C-8HE, a cosmetic type for hair and/or scalp surfaces, is **0.2 mm long (200 pm), which is painless because it is shorter than** normal. CIT-8, meaning collagen induction therapy, is a medical type, with a length of 0.5 mm, which allows collagen to be induced and consequently the skin to be remodelled. The MF-8, with a needle length of 1.5 mm, makes it possible to create wide microchannels with greater depths in the epidermis and dermis and simultaneously destroys scar collagen. MS-4, whose main feature is a smaller cylinder, with a length of 1 cm and a diameter of 2 cm, accounting for 4 circular rows of needles with a total of 96 needles, which is 1.5 mm long, is extremely relevant to the need to be used in places with greater penetration and precision, such as acne scars.

DERMA SEAL

These devices are made in miniature versions of other **dermarrollers,** and feature different needle sizes (0.2 to 3 mm) and 0.12 mm lengths, which are mainly useful for localised scars, such as varicella scars. It focuses on isolated scars, and being introduced with a vertical penetration allows infusion channels to be created in the skin, making it ideal for scars and wrinkles too.

DERMAPEN

Automated technology device in a unique pen format. It is an ergonomic device designed to use disposable needles, with a guide to more precisely adjust the length of needles with fractional mechanical resurgence. It has 9 to 12 needles organised in rows, is rechargeable and has a battery that can operate in two modes: a high speed mode (700 cycles per minute) and a low speed mode (412 cycles per minute) with vibrations similar to those of a stamp.

The biggest advantage of this device is that it can be reused on different patients, making it possible to discard the needles, and it is most useful for narrow areas of the nose, lip and eye contours, without damaging other areas. It is one of the most painless and cost-effective procedures, precisely because there is no reason to buy another one. This device was created to improve and overcome barrier applications such as variable pressure, with better penetration range.

FIGURA 2   Dermapen together with the charger

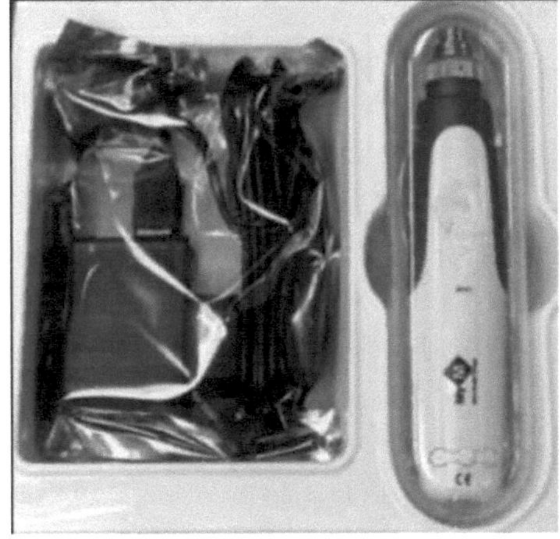

DERMAFRAC

Dermafrac is a technology that since its development has sought to unite several other forms of treatment in a single format, becoming the latest device to combine microneedling with microdermabrasion, deep tissue sorbent infusion and light-emitting iodine (LED). This innovation allows for better results in indications for skin ageing, sun damage, as well as deep acne, enlarged pores, divergent pigmentation, wrinkles, fine lines, hyperpigmentation and superficial scars.

The method used for this procedure can take approximately 45 minutes for the entire facial treatment when used in all four modalities. It has a great advantage because it is economical and less invasive, differing from other devices in that it does not produce downtime with pre-selected serums used in the infusion.

MICRO-NEEDLE DELIVERY SYSTEM

This needle delivery mechanism has the particularity of offering minimally invasive and painless resources for transmitting the transdermal drug, making it more useful in vaccines. The shape of the needles available can be solid and coated, dissolving hollow, swellable polymer microneedles synthesised by micro-manufacturing techniques. The main types of suitable material used to manufacture this mechanism can be silicon, metals in the same proportion as titanium, with natural or synthetic polymers and polysaccharides forming part of the essential microneedles.

Needles made from these solid materials allow for safer drug delivery by superficially piercing the skin before topical drug application, while soluble or biodegradable hollow needles deliver the drugs.

FRACTIONAL RADIOFREQUENCY MICRONEEDLING (MNFR)

This treatment perspective is one of the great promises, made through the amalgamation of micro-needles with the incidence of radiofrequency, penetrating the skin in a format that performs the isolation of the needles when penetrated into the skin, then releasing the radiofrequency directly from the tip of the needles through the thermal zones in the desired target that would be the dermal structures together with the glandular accessories, and not attacking the epidermis superimposed on the site.

Its methodology works over long periods of time that are predetermined according to the skin type, giving importance to the factors of neolastogenesis and neocollagenesis for long periods of time. The needles can or should be adjusted between 0.5 mm and 3.5 mm, with the need to focus on different places and layers of the dermis discreetly, the qualified professional can at this point adjust the power levels of the energy pulses, preventing future possible damage. The energy delivery system has a tip around it that can be disposable, with 49 micro-needles used in its energy delivery, which in some devices can be done with gold-plated needles. The MNRF is currently one of the pioneers for dark skins, as it does not reach the epidermis, guaranteeing good safety performance, especially in dark skins and indicated for scars, hyperhidrosis, rejuvenation and others.

LIGHT-EMITTING MICROPHONE DEVICE

The LED present in the mechanisms of microneedling devices are present in only a few places because they have only recently been launched. Their composition is a spill of titanium microneedles and LED lights, very effective for wrinkles and scars, but they still need to be explored extensively for use in other factors that damage the skin.

PRINCIPLE AND MECHANISM OF ACTION

The mechanism is basically based on micro-scarring, which is triggered from the moment the micro-needles penetrate the skin, which consequently causes easily controlled skin lesions, not damaging the epidermis, starting with the formation of these micro-injuries leading to small, short-lived bleeding, creating a cascade aimed at healing, releasing various growth factors with this process, such as platelet-derived growth factor, alpha and beta growth factors, proteins responsible for activating connective tissue and fibroblast-derived growth factors.

The needles act precisely on old scars already fixed in place, allowing a renewal of vascularisation, neovascularisation and neocllagenesis occurs with the migration and increase of fibroblasts, under the intercellular matrix, then a matrix of phobronectin is formed around the 5th day of the lesion's formation, determining the formation of collagen that results in the stiffening of the skin, persisting for up to a possible 7 years, in the form of type III collagen.

Neocollagenesis at a depth of between 5 and 600 pm is ideal for a needle 1.5 mm long, as in histological analyses of the skin it is possible to see that with four sessions or one month of cell reorganisation at the site there can be a 400% increase in collagen, as well as a deposition of elastin present mainly in post-operative patients, significant thickness of the spinous extract, cumites with typical characteristics in one year of post-operative patients and the bundles of fibres that were previously parallel in damaged skin forming into bundles of collagen fibres typically recognisable in their normal forms.

Proteins such as potassium and growth factors are released to the outside, causing a large migration of fibroblasts into the lesion, inducing significant collagen formation, and suddenly scars form in one direction as if these cells were migrating through a larger lesion.

The hyperpigmentation induced by microneedling is expressed by matrix metalloproteinase, and there is hypoploriferation of the keratinocytes reorganised after microneedling to improve cellular balance.

CHAPTER 4

Microneedling technique purpose

First presented by Orentreich and Orentreich (1995) under the name of subcision, the purpose of the microneedling technique is to produce collagen in the treatment of scars and rhytides. Desmond Fernandes (2006) created a device for percutaneous collagen induction therapy (CIT) and labelled it the "Dermaroller", from which year the technique began to spread around the world.

The equipment consists of a roller covered with fine surgical stainless steel or titanium alloy needles, which are various lengths in diameter.

This aesthetic device aims to stimulate collagen production through skin perforations that cause an inflammatory process. As a result, growth factors are released, which favour cell proliferation, especially fibroblasts, promoting the synthesis of supporting proteins.

The device is made of polyethylene material, cylindrical in shape, and contains stainless steel micro-needles in several rows, ranging from 0.25 mm to 2.5 mm. Injuries are classified as mild, moderate and deep, each related to the size of the needle used and the indications for each injury in each dysfunction.

In the process, micro-punctures are made on the skin, triggering a loss of skin integrity, with the aim of exchanging damaged collagen fibres for new ones. This results in the dissociation of keratinocytes and the release of cytokines, which generate vasodilation at the site, leading to the migration of keratinocytes to re-establish the damaged tissue. By rolling the equipment over the skin, microchannels are created and the formulations applied permeate very effectively and quickly.

The advantages of the procedure are the production of collagen without removing the epidermal layer; reduced healing time, and the risk of side effects is small compared to other techniques; the skin becomes more resistant and thicker, unlike ablative techniques, in which the resulting scar tissue is more subject to photodamage. The low cost compared to aesthetic procedures that require technologies with high financial investment.

The treatment is carried out at intervals of one to two months, and several sessions are needed to achieve the desired effect. The use of the dermaroller has been gaining ground worldwide, not only as a treatment for blemishes such as acne, but also as a rejuvenation method. The technique varies according to its approach, from the lightest to the heaviest, so its use should be carried out by a specialised professional in order to avoid aggravation.

15

Contraindications to microneedling are rare and severe forms of scarring, propensity to keloids, high phototypes, diabetes, pregnancy, cancer, warts, acute acne, herpes, solar erythema, rosacea, allergy to the metal or cosmetic used, vascular disease, bleeding disorder, neuromuscular disease and acute or chronic therapy with anticoagulants, anti-inflammatories and corticosteroids.

CHAPTER 5

Collagen production

WHAT IS COLLAGEN

In the development of pluricellular organisms, cells progressively form tissues, i.e. more specialised groups of cells. The space between one cell and another is filled by substances secreted by the cells themselves, which make up the extracellular matrix.

This matrix is a complex network made up of four major classes of macromolecules: collagens, proteoglycans, glycosaminoglycans and adhesive glycoproteins, which ensure a physical skeleton to support the tissue structure, configuring hydration and, consequently, the volume of the tissue, creating spaces for the transport of molecules, dynamic organisation and resistance to compressive forces. Among the macromolecules mentioned, we will study collagen, as well as its characteristics, importance and production.

Collagen is considered to be the largest class of insoluble fibrous protein found in the extracellular matrix and connective tissues and is also of fundamental importance in its constitution, as it is responsible for a large part of its physical properties. It contains peptide chains of the amino acids glycine, proline, lysine, hydroxylysine, hydroxyproline and alanine. These chains are arranged parallel to an axis, forming the collagen fibres, which provide strength and elasticity to the structure in which it is present. It can be referred to as a family of relative yet genetically different proteins whose main function is structural.

Collagen fibrils are formed by the polymerisation or triple helix interlacing of elongated molecular units called tropocollagen, consisting of three subunits (polypeptide chains) joined by hydrogen bridges (FIGURE 3). This protein structural configuration justifies the physical and biological properties of the collagen molecule: rigidity, solidity and stability.

Collagen can be found in a number of places in the body, including bones, tendons, cartilage, veins, skin, teeth, muscles and the stratum corneum of the eyes, in the connective tissues of the body as a whole and can contribute to the structural integrity of the tissues in which it is present. This protein, classified as being of animal origin, has the function of providing firmness to the skin, cartilage and, in general, to structures in our body that don't need bones as a means of providing support, but rather support.

However, as the years go by, at the beginning of adulthood itself, the body has a decrease in collagen levels, thus marking the period in which this collagen deficiency begins to be noticed, this event is due to a decrease in its production in the body, making it necessary to supplement it by external means in order to provide prevention of the early appearance of degenerative diseases as a result of a wrong diet.

CHARACTERISTICS OF COLLAGEN

The most important characteristic of hydrolysed collagen is its amino acid composition, providing a high level of glycine and proline, two essential amino acids for the stability and regeneration of cartilage. It therefore has beneficial effects on the body.

Collagen fibrils are formed by the polymerisation of elongated molecular units called tropocollagen, consisting of three subunits (polypeptide chains) arranged in a triple helix, joined by hydrogen bridges.

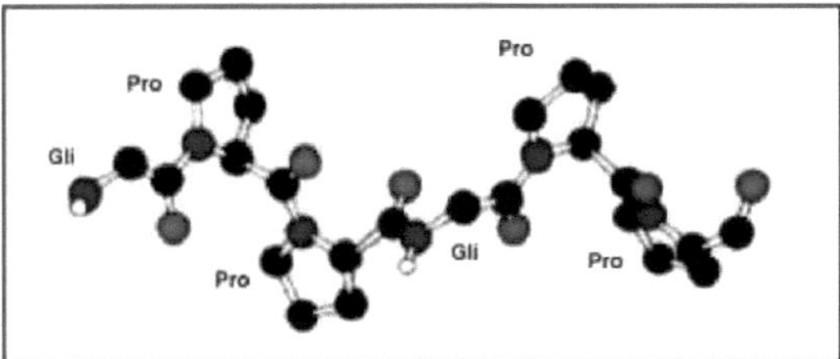

FIGURA 3   : Conformation of a single filament of the collagen triple helix.

29 different genetic types of collagen have been identified, many of which have unique characteristics and some of which have interrelated characteristics; however, all of them are formed by polypeptide subunits called chains. Of these, nine are frequently available, including Types I, II, III, IV, V and VII collagens,

IX, XI and XII and can be divided into two types of collagen: fibrillar and non-fibrillar collagens. Fibrillar types I, II and III form typical collagen fibrils with an axial periodicity of 67 nm and are the most abundant collagens.

Types I, II, III, V, X, XXIV and XXVII collagens line up in large extracellular fibrils and are referred to as fibril-forming collagens or fibrillar collagens.

Type I collagen is the most abundant and can be found in the skin, tendons, ligaments and bones. This collagen is a macromolecular protein made up of three **polypeptide chains (two a1 and one a2) that are helical in their** central **portion** and globular at the anemic and carboxylic ends.

In collagens I and II the tropocollagen molecules join together through hydrogen bridges, hydrophobic interactions and covalent bonds to form the fibrils

In type II (present in cartilage), fibrils are formed, but not fibres. Collagen IV, present in the basal membrane, does not form fibres or fibrils, but is organised in an interlacing within the basal membranes. In this collagen there is a peculiar association forming a complex weave and its structure is made up of a triple helix of two **a1 (Type IV) and one a2 (Type IV) polypeptide chains.**

Type VI forms distinct microfibrils and Type VII forms anchoring fibrils. Fibrillar-associated collagens are short structures that connect collagen fibrils to each other and to other components of the extracellular matrix. Types IX, XII, XIV, XIX, XX and XXI collagens belong to this group.

IMPORTANCE OF COLLAGEN

Collagen is important because it fulfils various functions in the human body, the most important of which are the maintenance and reconstitution of the skin, bones, cartilaginous tissues and the extracellular matrix. However, there are many others, such as keeping tissue cells together and strengthening them, it is responsible for healing and/or regeneration in the event of continuity damage or surgery, it helps to moisturise the body and is thought to be linked to the human ageing process, especially signs of skin ageing such as wrinkles and facial furrows.

It also has high elasticity and is considered the most important functional protein in the body.

In addition, some diseases are related to this protein, in fact to its decrease or absence. These are collectively called collagenoses or collagen diseases, which are characterised by a group of autoimmune and inflammatory diseases that damage the body's connective tissue (tissue made up of fibres such as collagen) and correspond to pathologies that bring with them autoimmune characteristics with a high potential for affecting organs such as the lungs, among others. They can also include rheumatoid arthritis, progressive systemic sclerosis, systemic lupus erythematosus, dermatopolymyositis, mixed connective tissue disease and Sjogren's syndrome, direct and indirect inguinal hernia and some rare forms of muscular dystrophy.

Collagen is also important for maintaining the tone and firmness of the dermis. In order for this protein to be synthesised properly, there needs to be synergism between vitamin C and an adequate intake of proteins that provide the amino acids that make up collagen, as vitamin C is directly linked to the synthesis of collagen and glycosaminoglycans.

COLLAGEN PRODUCTION

The process of collagen synthesis begins with the transcription of genes and subsequent translation of messenger RNA by the ribosomes (organelles responsible for making polypeptide chains) of the rough endoplasmic reticulum (RER). In the lumen of the RER is procollagen, which undergoes successive hydroxylation and glycosylation processes on its amino acids lysine and proline, forming the triple helix. The triple helix is sent to the Golgi Complex (the organelle responsible for producing secretory vesicles) and is then secreted into the extracellular matrix (ECM). When secreted into the extracellular space, the tropocollagen molecules assemble into higher order polymers such as collagen fibrils. These fibrils often aggregate into bundles several micrometres long, called collagen fibres. During fibrillogenesis, proteoglycans guide and stabilise the formation and maturation of collagen fibrils.

The collagen molecule is 280 nm long, with a molecular mass of 300,000 Da, stabilised by hydrogen bridges and intermolecular bonds. The amino acid sequence in collagen is generally a tripeptide unit, glycine-X-proline or glycine-X-hydroxyproline, where the X can be any of the 20 standard amino acids. Each collagen molecule can have up to three different chains, which join together to form procollagen

The process of producing this protein occurs mainly during the preparation, regeneration and development of embryonic tissue. Collagen molecules are secreted by fibroblasts (the constituent cell of connective tissue and its function is to form the amorphous fundamental substance) in the form of soluble procollagen, which has on each of its sides globular peptide structures containing nitrogen (N-) and carbon (C-) terminals.

Procollagen is secreted into the vesicles formed in the Golgi apparatus and then secreted into the extracellular matrix (Figure 2). In the extracellular matrix, C- and N-peptidases act to cleave the two globular structures attached to the ends of the procollagen. The action of these enzymes is necessary to start the process of fibrillogenesis (collagen production), as these globular structures attached to procollagen occupy a large space around the molecule.

Thus, the cleavage process is necessary for the formation of tropocollagen, which begins to join with other tropocollagen molecules to form fibrils. The tropocollagen molecules come together in a twisted conformation by means of side-by-side associations, stabilised primarily by hydrophobic and electrostatic interactions.

The molecular structure of collagen is relatively simple and it is insoluble in water due to the high concentration of hydrophobic amino acids that make up the inside and outside of the protein on the surface. It is an exception to the rule that hydrophobic groups must be hidden inside the protein molecule. The hydrophobic core therefore contributes less to the structural stability of the molecule, while covalent bonds play a particularly important role.

CHAPTER 6

Healing in the microneedling process

Microneedling is a technique widely used in aesthetic procedures to treat and/or improve the appearance of the skin. It is widely used for facial rejuvenation, to treat acne scars, stretch marks and alopecia. This procedure is currently gaining a lot of ground, as it is a low-invasive and very effective technique. Microneedling is carried out using a device known as a roller, a roller-shaped piece of equipment made up of small, fine needles ranging from 0.5 to 3.0 mm in length and 0.1 to 0.8 mm in diameter. These needles are sterile and are used to make micro-holes in the epidermis, the most superficial layer of the skin.

These small holes, which do not damage or deform the epidermis, stimulate the synthesis of collagen in the area, thus improving its appearance, as well as providing a gateway for the active ingredients used in the procedure, which penetrate to the deeper layers of the skin and enhance the effect of the treatment. In addition to the technique itself, which stimulates collagen synthesis at the site, offering a better arrangement for the collagen fibres and encouraging the creation of new vessels, it is also important to use certain cosmetological actives that will act in the process and enhance the expected result.

The process of skin healing is characterised as the replacement of damaged tissue with vascularised tissue, unlike the process of regeneration, which only consists of the recovery of lost tissue, restoring the skin to its previous characteristics. Healing takes place in three stages. The first of these is the inflammatory phase, which is caused by small lesions in the skin during the microneedling procedure. This inflammation can occur at the moment of the lesion and last around 72 hours. The inflammation caused is of paramount importance in the treatment, as it triggers a series of physiological mechanisms that will act to favour the desired tissue repair. The small lesion generates cell proliferation and an increase in cell metabolism at the site, causing the release of some elements, such as blood, containing plasma and platelets that will act in blood coagulation, forming a fibrin barrier that will act as protection, making it impossible for microorganisms to enter.

The platelets that have been released by the injured endothelium promote the coagulation cascade, dispensing granules that contain certain substances, such as platelet growth factors, fibroblast and epidermal growth factors, thromboxanes and prostaglandins. These factors promote chemotaxis, leading neutrophils to the injured site through vasodilation and increased vascular permeability. Neutrophils are the first cells to arrive at the wound site, they act by adhering to the endothelium wall via membrane receptors and are largely responsible for producing free radicals that will act to destroy bacteria, progressively being replaced by macrophages. These in turn actively contribute to the secretion of cytokines and growth factors, causing angiogenesis and the synthesis of extracellular matrix.

The second phase is proliferation, in which there is an increase in fibroblasts that secrete substances that are very important in the healing process, such as collagen and elastin. The induction of collagen occurs through the disaggregation of keratinocytes by abrasion of the skin, which enables the release of cytokines that will cause dermal vasodilation. Fibroblasts are responsible for synthesising and secreting polypeptide chains, which are called pro-collagen. Through the action of certain enzymes, pro-collagen gives rise to collagen, forming the fibres that give elasticity and firmness to the tissue. Collagen synthesis is regulated by two important components: TGF-0 and AP-1, the former a growth factor and the latter a protein-1 activator.

Fibroblasts and endothelial cells are the main components of this phase. The PDGF factor is responsible for the proliferation and activation of fibroblasts, which will be stimulated to produce collagen by the release of the TGF-0 factor. As well **as acting on** fibroblasts, PDGF is also responsible for matrix synthesis and chemotaxis. Other factors such as epidermal factor, transforming factor alpha, transforming factor beta and fibroblast factor act respectively to stimulate epithelialisation, angiogenesis, matrix synthesis and cell proliferation. They all work together in harmony for an effective healing process, reorganising the collagen fibres and acquiring an appropriate appearance.

This is followed by the remodelling or maturation phase, which consists of an organisation of the collagen fibres. There is a slow exchange of type III collagen for type I collagen, which lasts for 5 to 7 years. This exchange is carried out by fibroblasts and leukocytes that secrete collagenases, a substance that plays a very important role in lysing the old collagen matrix. The remodelling process is of great importance and is characterised by a balance between lysis of the old matrix and increased production of the new collagen matrix. This whole sequence of factors enables the formation of more fibrous tissue, giving the skin a more uniform appearance.

Collagen is the most abundant and important protein in this process, formed by a dense and dynamic network, the result of its constant modification by the process of deposition and resorption. It gives the skin elasticity and firmness and is physiologically deposited in the dermis in the form of organised collagen fibres. It has at least 19 types of collagen, the most common of which are found in the skin, with a percentage of 85% to 90% and 8% to 11% being type I collagen and type III collagen, respectively.

The healing process carried out using the microneedling technique is substantially faster and the side effects are minimal compared to other aesthetic procedures. As a result, microneedling has become a very relevant and effective option because, in addition to its low cost, the results are very satisfactory, promoting a great improvement in the appearance of scars on the skin as well as in problems that require greater vascularisation.

CHAPTER 7

Microbiological risks of reusing the dermaroller with the main bacteria that affect the skin and mucosa

STAPHYLOCOKS

The genus **Staphylococcus is** responsible for numerous bacterial infections in humans and can be divided into two large groups based on the coagulase enzyme produced. The first group is known as coagulase-positive **Staphylococcus, which is** represented by **Staphylococcus aureus.** The second group, known as **Staphylococcus coagulase** negative (SCN), is represented by numerous strains: **S. epidermidis, S. haemolyticus, S. saprophyticus, S. lugdunensis, S. cohnii, S. schleiferi, S. simulans, S. hominis, S. warneri, S. capitis, S. caprae and S. xylosus.**

Staphylococcus is one of the pathogenic elements that forms part of the normal microbiota of human beings and is characterised as transient or resident without causing any symptoms. It is detected in various parts of the body, such as the nasal cavities, which are the main reservoir of the bacteria. Staph infections can be caused by the individual's own bacteria, which are called endogenous infections, or they can be caused by samples obtained from other patients or healthy carriers, which is known as cross-infection, through airborne contact, i.e. indirectly, or by direct contact, due to the presence of a patient or carrier.

Staphylococci are mesophilic microorganisms with a growth temperature of between 7 and 48.8°C. They can produce heat-resistant enterotoxins at temperatures between 10 and 46°C, with an optimum temperature of between 40 and 45°C. The ideal pH for development is between 7 and 7.5, but it is possible to multiply in foods ranging from 4.2 to 9.3. **Staphylococci** are a group of microorganisms that have the ability to multiply and survive in a certain amount of sodium chloride at concentrations of up to 15% and the production of enterotoxin occurs in salt concentrations of up to 10%, which is the cause of transmission through food and can favour high levels of poisoning.

Staphylococci are bacteria that are sensitive to high temperatures, as well as to disinfectants and antiseptic products, but some microorganisms can remain alive in dry rooms for an extended period of time. **Staphylococcus aureus** is considered to be the most virulent and common bacterial species of the genus. The endogenous spread of this bacterium is the most constant and is responsible for many infections, in response to the presence of **staphylococcus** on the human flora. However, exogenous spread can occur where the bacteria can be transported to a vulnerable individual through direct contact or by fomites. It is therefore necessary for healthcare professionals to use appropriate techniques such as hand washing, thus preventing the spread of microorganisms to patients.

S. aureus has expanded a number of virulence devices and tactics to evade the human immune system, encompassing a sequence of surface proteins, secreted enzymes and toxins that deteriorate the membrane by cytolytic action. These devices can cause anything from a simple infection such as pimples, boils and impetigo, to more complex infections such as meningitis, periocarditis, bacteraemia and toxic shock syndrome.

In the mid-1940s and 1950s, infections caused by **S. aureus** were treated with penicillin (methicillin), which was a powerful agent against the bacterial cell wall. However, microorganisms soon developed that were resistant to antimicrobials with a beta-lactam ring. For this reason, a set of penicillins was developed in the laboratory that had an altered beta-lactam ring and were therefore effective against these bacteria.

At the beginning of the 1970s, strains of **S. aureus** with resistance to methicillin, recognised by the acronym MRSA (methicillin-resistant **S. aureus**), began to appear, as well as resistance to other beta-lactams, such as cephalosporins. MRSA micro-organisms have the ability to spread rapidly, especially in hospital environments, thus limiting the demand for antibiotic treatment for infections caused by these strains to glycopeptides such as teicoplanin and vancomycin.

In places that require more care, the extent of MRSAs in relation to infections caused by **S. aureus** increased unusually between 1974 and 2014. The presence of this strain in communities has been gaining ground in a similar way, thus representing a significant public health burden. Thus, the emergence of resistant microorganisms such as MRSA requires an immediate search for new antibiotics.

Staphylococci are Gram- and catalase-positive cocci, about 0.5 to 1.5 pm in diameter, without motility, non-sporulated. They can be arranged in various ways, ranging from isolated, in pairs, in small chains, or grouped disproportionately, with the appearance of a bunch of grapes, due to cell fractionation, which takes place in different planes. Numerous physiological, morphological and chemical characteristics co-operate in the virulence of **S. aureus.**

These microorganisms carry a polysaccharide capsule that forms the outermost layer of the cell wall. Eleven capsular serotypes of **S. aureus have** been found, with serotypes 6 and 7 being those related to infections in humans. The capsule can make bacterial phagocytosis impossible by hiding the opsonins, thus increasing virulence and the ability to invade tissue, as well as the bloodstream, via a peripheral focus. The external region of the vast majority of **S. aureus** strains contains the coagulation factor, bound coagulase, which binds to fibrinogen and converts it into insoluble fibrin, making it an important virulence factor.

The membrane of bacteria is made up of a complex containing proteins, lipids and a small amount of carbohydrates. It acts as an osmotic barrier for the cell and provides an anchor for cellular respiratory and biosynthetic enzymes. These are some of the physiological, morphological and chemical characteristics that allow **S. aureus to** invade the host, escape its defences, multiply and settle, thus inducing the manifestation of diseases. The pathogenicity of this strain is due to its virulence factors and its high resistance to various antimicrobials. Both factors effectively help bacterial colonisation at points of infection.

Numerous diseases caused by **S. aureus** are caused by the production of toxins, such as scalded skin syndrome, heat shock syndrome and food poisoning, while several diseases result from the multiplication of microorganisms, resulting in the appearance of abscesses and the demolition of tissues, such as endocarditis, skin infection, pneumonia, osteomyelitis, empyema and septic atritis.The most common analyses for diagnosing MRSA are the use of appropriate culture media and subsequent **screening** for bacterial cultures using oxacillin discs, which are favoured because they are more stable during storage. However, the use of molecular techniques is faster and more sensitive.

Staphylococcus aureus has methods of defence against certain drugs. Strains with abundant resistance, such as those of **S. aureus,** are more commonly found in hospital environments and can cause possible consequences such as clinical and epidemiological problems. These resistances end up limiting therapeutic alternatives, as well as extending the time it takes to treat infections.

Medical resources that support and monitor simple bodily functions collaborate greatly in the success of medical treatments. However, by overcoming defence barriers, these resources facilitate the entry of microorganisms into fluids and tissues that are regularly sterile, leading to an increase in infections in hospital and laboratory environments, mainly by MRSA2. Although there are new antimicrobial agents, such as linezolid, vancomycin remains the standard form of therapy for treating infections caused by these multidrug-resistant types.

Linezolid, which belongs to the oxazolidinone class, has been recognised by the US Food and Drug Administration for skin infections, as well as soft tissue and MRSA pneumonia. In clinical terms, its effectiveness is similar to vancomycin, with rare resistance. However, linezolid is expensive and has substantial toxicity potential, including myelosuppression, peripheral neuropathy, lactic acidosis and optic neuritis, so this drug should be saved for more serious infections when other oral drugs are not as susceptible.
STREPTOCOS

Brown, in 1919, observed the heterogeneity of **streptococci** in animals and humans, determining the first classification order of these bacteria into a, P **and y based on haemolysis patterns that were verified on plates containing** blood agar **culture medium.** Thus, *streptococcus* colonies that generate a clear halo around them, due to the total lysis of red blood cells, were characterised as P-hemolytic. Most strains of *streptococci that are* pathogenic to humans are part of this haemolysis pattern, such as *S. pyogenes, S. agalactiae and others.*

Strains of *streptococci* that generate partial haemolysis show a greenish, shiny colour around the colony, and are characterised as a-haemolysis, as they show this colour exclusively in culture, and are established as the *viridans* group. This group includes several species of *streptococcus* and *pneumococcus* that occupy the respiratory tree and gastrointestinal tract, as well as being the main culprits in heart valve infections. Colonies that do not show haemolysis are characterised as y or non-hemolytic, which rarely cause infections in humans.

Streptococci are Gram-positive, ovoid or spherical bacteria, most of which do not have motility, their diameter varies from 1 to 2jim, **they** are **catalase negative and** are normally facultative anaerobes. They are presented in chains when found in liquid media and commonly in pairs in vitro. They belong to the *Streptococcaceae* family, of the *Streptococcus* genus, which has 21 different species. Because of their heterogeneity, these microorganisms require different laboratory identification processes to specify their characterisation, analysing the pattern of haemolysis, antigenic composition, growth characteristics and biochemical interactions.

In the mid-1990s, Rebecca Lancefield demonstrated an innovative classification system using antigenic constituents of the bacterial cell wall. Using specific sera, she tested their precipitation reactions and thus identified different serogroups (A, B, C, D..., K) of P-hemolytic streptococci. Subsequently, it was also found that some **a and y haemolytic** strains **may possess** group-specific antigens.

The cellular structure of **streptococci** consists of capsules, a cell wall and a cytoplasmic membrane. The capsules of serogroups A and C are made up of hyaluronic acid, which gives the colony a mucoid appearance. This envelope of the streptococcus leads to phagocytosis by polymorphonuclear leukocytes and macrophages and is therefore characterised as a virulence factor. The cell wall is the element that is related to pathogenicity. It is made up of various surface protein antigens on the outermost part: proteins M, T and R. Below these is the carbohydrate C and the innermost part is made up of peptidoglycan, which is responsible for rigidity. The cytoplasmic or cell membrane is found on the inner wall of the cell wall, is thin, lipoprotein and contains antigens. **Streptococci** that lose their cell wall are covered by this membrane, which, by the way, becomes weakened and resistant to penicillin and other P-lactams.

Serogroup A *haemolytic Streptococcus* is Gram positive and can be detected on the skin of healthy humans and in the upper airways. It is estimated that 15 to 20 per cent of the population carry the bacteria, which can fluctuate among school-age children, depending on where you live, taking into account the season and environmental humidity. Invasive infections
by group A *Streptococcus,* have an incidence of between 1.5 and 6.8 cases per 100,000 inhabitants, according to Canadian, Swedish and American data. The most common complications are osteomyelitis, arthritis, septic shock, pneumonia, meningitis, necrotising fasciitis and empyema.

The annual incidence of group A **Streptococcus** in industrialised countries is very high. This incidence is three times higher among the elderly over the age of 70, and the older the person, the higher the incidence. The elderly are also shown to have the highest mortality rates, with studies considering clinical syndromes showing that age favours and increases the risk of death, regardless of the strain of serogroup A **Streptococcus.**

In 1980, there was a sustained worldwide increase in the occurrence of serious invasive infections caused by serogroup A **Streptococci, the** main ones being **Streptococcus pyogenes.** The reasons for the occurrence of group A **Streptococcus** diseases are completely unclear, but a fractional explanation may be the common dispersal of a colony of serotype M1T1 strains. The strains considered to be invasive M1T1 present genes that are associated with bacteriophages, encoding virulence factors, such as the exotoxin SpeA and secreted DNase Sda1 (SdaD2), both of which are correlated with the pathogenicity of group A **Streptococcus** in model systems.

The detection of **Streptococcus pyogenes in** culture media, carried out specifically in the laboratory, shows optimal growth on media such as blood agar. Immediately after incubation for 24 hours at 37°C, **white colonies of 1 to 2 mm** can be seen with **large halos of** p-hemolysis. This is due to the total haemolysis of the erythrocytes present in the culture medium. The supposed identification is made using the classification described by Lancefield, which differentiates the species of p-hemolytic *streptococci*. This technique is based on the differences in immunological polysaccharides found in the cell wall (Group A, B, C, F and G) or in lipoprotein acids (Group D).

A large proportion of the streptococci isolated from human infections that agglutinate in serum A of the Lancefield classification represent the *Streptococcuspyogenes* strain. It is precisely for this reason that these strains are categorised as group A *streptococci*. Rarely, however, some Streptococcus species, *such* as *S. dysgalactia and S. anginosusc collected from* humans, can also present the A-carbohydrate. In these cases, if not subjected to other techniques, the species may be incorrectly identified.

The detection of vulnerability to bacitracin is also frequently used for testing, with the intention of differentiating **S. pyogenes** species **from** other strains of P-hemolytic **streptococci.** Many strains of **S.** *pyogenes* are sensitive to this antimicrobial, although some species have been reported to be resistant. The most widely used option for treating bacterial infections is the administration of antimicrobials. Since the beginning of their use, several cases of resistance and the spread of numerous associated mechanisms have been reported. Given that the antibiotic of choice can be decisive in the course of the infection, it is important to regularly monitor the resistance levels of the antimicrobial treatment method adopted, so that it is the most appropriate.

Pathogenic bacteria in their common state show changes in virulence and disease potential among isolates. *Staphylococcus aureus isolates* from the United States have emerged as a predominant cause of skin infections, and these isolates show enhanced virulence factor expression. In addition to the fact that the pathogenic bacterium is of great concern to public health, due to possible failures in therapeutic treatment and the withdrawal of preventative regimes, there is often a lack of information on the molecular mechanisms that give rise to the variations. Possible mechanisms include the acquisition of genes behind the pathogen's variation, which are transferred via horizontal genes. The loss of genes through genome reduction or the modulation of systems that regulate and lead to changes in expression patterns.

Group A *Streptococcus* is characteristic of humans, a pathogen that causes infections ranging from mild to severe. Group A strains are divided **into serotypes based on sequences at the 5' end of the M coding protein.** Some serotypes of group A **Streptococcus are** randomly associated with disease manifestations. As in the case of strains with M3 serotypes, which are associated with unusual and severe invasive infections, with a high lethality rate. The M18 serotype protein is associated with colonies that cause outbreaks of acute rheumatic fever and the M28 serotype is associated with strains that cause cases of puerperal sepsis.

Although more than five decades have passed since these associations were distinguished, the molecular basis continues to be exposed. When group A *Streptococcus* strains show gene variation, primarily the result of integrated bacteriophages is different, as none are identical to their serotype of origin. Since the core genomes of all group A strains are highly conserved and harbour a range of common virulence factors, it has been assumed that the differential regulation of these virulence factors is the centre of attention in most group A serotype associations.

CHAPTER 8

Skin diseases caused by bacteria

Human beings have bacteria that are able to protect them from certain infectious agents, and therefore pathogens. These are called bacteria that make up the normal microbiota. However, there are others that trigger skin diseases. Among these bacteria are the main ones: **Staphylococcus aureus** and **Streptococcus**.

Each of them is capable of producing different diseases and complications, and **S. aureus** is also directly and indirectly related to the ingestion of contaminated food, such as untreated milk or milk that has not undergone the pasteurisation process, due to the lack of sanitary control of the food ingested by human beings.

STAPHYLOCOCCUS AUREUS

S. auerus is related to its high resistance to antibiotics, as it is a highly pathogenic bacterium. In terms of morphology, they are gram-positive cocci with positive coagulase and are bhemolytic.

As it is a mesophilic microorganism, i.e. it survives at temperatures that are not too low, it can, however, grow at thermophilic temperatures, characterised by its high thermal resistance, which makes it capable of surviving temperature-based treatments, such as pasteurisation, in order to reduce its contamination of the most widely used foodstuff, milk.

Pathogenesis occurs through the enterotoxins it produces, which can cause heat shock and various allergic reactions. The main symptoms of **staphylococcal** gastroenteritis (food poisoning caused by **Staphylococcus aureus**) are nausea, vomiting, diarrhoea followed by abdominal pain, among other symptoms. Depending on the individual's susceptibility, it can progress to more severe conditions.

With the use of serological tests, it is possible to identify 7 (seven) types of toxins produced by **Staphylococcus, known as** staphylococcal enterotoxins: A, B, C1, C2, C3,D, E, G, H, and I. The one most commonly identified in cases of infection is enterotoxin A.

In recent decades, researchers and health professionals have faced problems when it comes to bacterial resistance. Some bacteria have the ability to resist antibiotics such as penicillin. **Staphylococcus aureus** is currently the most notorious for being the most resistant pathogen when it comes to infections, and is the main hospital-acquired infection. As mentioned above, it has a high degree of resistance, making treatment with certain antibiotics ineffective.

It is known that **S. aureus** is part of the human microbiota (skin and nasal cavities), called the normal microbiota, and that the infections caused by it range from simple infections such as boils to more complex, severe and more diagnosed infections, such as skin diseases: Cutaneous Botryomycosis.

FURUCTION

A simple infection caused by S aureus, a furuncle is characterised by the bacteria entering the hair follicles, causing oedema, which can lead to the presence of nodules (multiple in one area), with a reddish appearance (as a result of the toxins they release), with a hardened texture, and almost always the presence of pus, with the main symptom being a high temperature and pain in the affected area. The size of the pus can vary, as it correlates with the depth at which the battery lodges in the tissues.

This infection mainly affects adults because it is an ingrown hair. It can cause scars. The main sites are the buttocks, legs and thighs, as these are the places most susceptible to this type of infection. This is also a consequence of the amount of hair, as it is a disease that affects the patient's hair follicles. However, it is important to emphasise that any part of the body can be infected by this pathogen (**S. aureus** bacteria).

In order to detect the disease, the most commonly requested test is a bacterial culture, which serves to clarify all possible doubts.

The methodology used for the test is to collect the sample using a sterile swab, where it will be deposited in the appropriate culture medium for the bacteria.

As with any disease caused by bacteria, treatment will be carried out with appropriate antibiotics (systemic) for the pathology.

CUTANEOUS BOTRYOMYCOSIS

It is characterised by an infection caused by bacteria, thus called a chronic bacterial infection. As well as affecting the skin, it can also affect the subcutaneous tissue and viscera, with a granulomatous and suppurative presentation, where a purulent secretion can be drained from the skin lesion and yellowish-white grains can be found (Mycetoma and Actinomycosis). This process of grains is still undefined, but there is an imbalance between host and parasite (antigen-antibody reaction).

The lesions may be multiple, single or pleomorphic, resembling nodules, abscesses or cysts. There may also be ulcers. They are usually located in the following regions: head, arms, legs and genitals, including male and female.

This infection was previously known to be caused by fungi (1884), hence the name Botryomycosis. Today, as it is an infection caused by bacteria, it has been given the appropriate names: Actinophytosis Staphylococcus, Bacterial Pseudomatosis, and Granular Bacteriosis.

Described by Bollinguer in 1870 thanks to the observation of lesions followed by complications after horses were castrated. However, it wasn't until 1913 that a researcher called Opie made it possible to describe the disease in humans. And in 1919, Magrou reported 4 (four) cases in which the main etiological agent was **Staphylococcus aureus.** However, in 1959 winslow proposed a review of the disease, in which 46 human cases were evaluated and the disease was classified as cutaneous and visceral infections.

The pathogenesis of the disease is currently unclear, but it may be related to the reduced virulence capacity of certain agents. It may also be due to a change in cellular immunity, which reduces the presence of T lymphocytes, further facilitating the infectious process.

Patients who are more susceptible to infection are: patients with diabetes mellitus, lung diseases such as pneumonia, among others.

The treatment of this infection is carried out firstly by identifying the etiological agent. This can be done by direct examination, culture of the secretion in the lesion and then an antibiogram. When the disease worsens, the lesions should be excised surgically or drained.

STREPTOCOS

Streptococci are facultative anaerobic bacteria that grow predominantly in atmospheric air and characteristically develop in chains (diplococci) when growing in broth media. Since the pathogens have various aspects that aid their virulence, the human skin and mucosa are the only reservoirs for group A **streptococcus** bacteria. **Streptococcus Pyogenes is** a group A **streptococcus** (GAS) and can be responsible for causing infections of varying degrees.

NON-BULLOUS IMPETIGO

Impetigo is the most common bacterial skin infection in childhood and affects both sexes equally. It can classically present as a bullous infection caused by *Staphylococus aureus* and a non-bullous infection caused by *haemolytic Streptococus,* but infections can be mixed. Some of the risk factors are poor hygiene, crowds, dermatological diseases that serve as a gateway and trauma to the skin (for example, microneedling during the use of a dermaroller).

Non-bullous impetigo is the most common form and usually begins with small red papules, rapidly developing into small pus-filled lesions (pustules), which burst and form golden crusted lesions. These lesions usually affect the face. Bullous impetigo presents vesiculobullous lesions caused by detachment of the epidermis, these blisters usually rupture and are covered by haematomeliceric crusts.

Treatment for these infections can be local, carried out through cleaning, the use of potassium permanganate or 3% boric water, with the use of local antibiotics: mupirocin 2% or fusidic acid and neomycin, and in the case of extensive lesions, systemic antibiotics are used: cephalexin, amoxicillin associated with clavulanic acid, cefaclor or clindamycin. Currently, penicillins and erythromycin are not the first choice of health professionals, as there is a possibility of resistance by methicillin-resistant strains of staphylococci.

ERISIPELLA and CELLULITIS

Erysipelas can be caused by group A p-hemolytic *Streptococci* (the most common cause of severe soft tissue infection in healthy individuals) and more rarely by *Staphylococus aureus*. It is a different type of cutaneous cellulitis, superficial, where there is marked involvement of the lymphatic vessels of the dermis. Cellulitis is an infectious process that affects the deep dermis and subcutaneous tissue, but the distinction between infected and uninfected tissue is not always clear. In the more common erysipelas, the area of inflammation stands out with a relief, indicating a different demarcation between the involved and normal tissue.

Even though the two conditions, erysipelas and cellulitis, when typical, can be easily distinguished, there can be variability in tissue involvement, making the differentiation not always so clear. Both conditions show local signs of inflammation (erythema, oedema, heat and pain) and, in most cases, fever and leucocytosis, while lymphangitis and/or lymphadenitis are also common. Cellulitis can also be caused by other bacteria and even some fungi.

In its normal function, the skin plays an important role in defence against a variety of pathogens. Cutaneous infection often arises as a result of a rupture of the epidermis and takes hold through the invasion of the pathogen into the dermis and subcutaneous tissue, so inflammatory mechanisms are activated in response to the invasion, and an area of the body distant from the affected area may be the entry point, making it not apparent in some cases, and local or distant foci of infection become less obvious. The entry point for cellulitis can be any mucocutaneous site or, rarely, via the haematogenous route to the loose tissues.

The normal microbiota of the skin is very important because if it is eradicated or diminished, some pathogenic species can proliferate and cause an infection. Once established, this infection spreads through tissue spaces and cleavage planes by the action of hyaluronidases, fibrinolysins and lecithinases. In addition, lymphatic and blood vessels are likely to be invaded, resulting in lymphangitis, lymphadenitis, bacteraemia and septicaemia.

Usually in the first episode of cellulitis, it can lead to impairment of the lymphatic vessels and predisposition to recurrent cellulitis, chronic lymphoedema and elephantiasis.

CUTANEOUS SMALL VESSEL VASCULITIS

Vasculitis is considered to be an inflammatory process that causes functional and structural damage to the vessel wall. This process is mediated by the immune system and can be classified as neutrophilic, lymphocytic and granulomatous according to the type of cells that predominate in the inflammatory agent of the process, as well as the location or size of the vessels. Necrotising vasculitis is characterised by rupture of the vessel wall associated with fibrinoid necrosis, and its histopathological expression is leucocytoclastic vasculitis.

Leukocytoclastic vasculitis begins after the deposition of immunocomplexes in the wall of the post-capillary venules of the dermis, which can be influenced by factors such as: hydrostatic pressure, turbulent blood flow in the terminal circulation of the skin, efficiency of the tissue macrophage system, platelet release of histamine and serotonin, and activation of the fibrinolytic system. The immune complexes present in the circulation interact with the endothelium, activating the endothelial cells, which causes the release of high levels of tissue plasminogen activator, which initiates the activation of the fibrinolytic system.

For a definitive diagnosis of necrotising vasculitis, elements such as leucocytoclasia and fibrinoid necrosis must be observed, but the characteristics that can be observed in the histopathological examination depend on the location of the lesion and also on how long it has been biopsied. When the process of vasculitis is already in the late stages, there may be pathogenic mechanisms other than those described and not yet fully understood, which determine the evolution of the process to a lymphocytic cutaneous infiltrate.

Vasculitis is generally divided into two groups: cutaneous small vessel vasculitis and necrotising large vessel vasculitis. This division takes into account clinical, etiopathogenic and histopathological aspects, although there is no worldwide consensus on their classification. The size of the blood vessel is related to its depth in the layers of the skin, because the deeper the location, the larger the diameter of the vessel. Small vessels are represented by capillaries, post-capillary venules and non-muscular arterioles.

less than 50pm in diameter and are preferentially found in the superficial **papillary dermis.**

Medium calibre vessels have a diameter of between 50 and 150pm and are located in the deep reticular dermis. Those with a **diameter greater than 150pm are not** found in the skin, so the typical skin biopsy will no longer be suitable for investigating vasculitis in medium calibre vessels. Other options are deep punch biopsy or deep surgical biopsy.

Vasculitis can be caused by various agents, including drugs, chemicals, food allergens, protozoan infections, viruses and bacteria. Bacterial infection can be caused by group A beta-haemolytic **Streptococcus, Staphylococcus aureus and Mycobacterium leprae.** When caused by infection, it can lead to certain symptoms (pseudovasculitis), such as infective endocarditis, septic vasculitis (septic vasculopathy) and Lucio's phenomenon.

CHAPTER 9

Biosecurity

Biosafety is a functional and operational system; it is a set of behaviours of great importance in health services, not because it provides measures to control contamination, but for the safety of health care staff and users. It also plays an essential role in promoting health awareness in the communities in which it operates, regarding the importance of prevention in the handling and disposal of toxic waste and contaminants and in controlling occupational risks. It is an evolving system that does not include a conclusion in its nomenclature and must therefore be constantly updated and monitored, offering immediate responses to the appearance of more resident and virulent microorganisms. The important objective of complying with biosafety regulations is to provide health professionals and institutions with the means to increase their activities with appropriate safety, both for the specialist and for the environment or community.

Biosafety is an element that must be respected in order for health professionals to carry out their activities and thus reduce the health risks for users and professionals who carry out the practices. There are two sides to biosafety: one related to handling and studying embryonic stem cells, which fulfils legal biosafety; and the other, biosafety used in hospitals, universities and doctor's surgeries, among other establishments. Developing a close relationship with various areas and disciplines of science, such as labour and health legislation. Its wide-ranging characteristics consider the prevention of health and the environment in the sense of preserving life.

It is essential to analyse what constitutes a health risk. This analysis will proceed in different ways, because each risk has its own characteristics, and is exposed to a greater or lesser degree of intensity, or magnitude, based on the conditions conducive to its verification. Once the severity of the risks has been assessed, prevention activities are organised, applying biosafety measures. The insecurity and risks of pathological infections that accompany today's population have put health systems to the test, changing society's international health framework. This has led to the development of a comprehensive approach to health and the relevance of interdisciplinary practices to understanding problems.

The use of biosafety standards is necessary for the growth of health safety techniques. The term biosafety appeared in the 1970s in the United States. With the emergence of biotechnology and the urgent need to formulate safety standards for procedures in laboratories where genetic samples would be manipulated. In 1980, the first biosafety manuals appeared. Over time, human beings have endeavoured to transform materials free of microorganisms.

Sanitary surveillance is responsible for distributing activities that can eliminate, reduce or prevent health risks. It is also responsible for interfering in health problems such as asepsis, sterilisation and the disposal of aesthetic materials and instruments that pose a risk of contamination by infectious agents to beauty professionals and clients. It is therefore the responsibility of health surveillance to monitor circumstances during these activities and to determine biosafety standards, preventing the reuse of aesthetic materials and instruments that can carry infectious agents and cause serious dermatological lesions, which is therefore an irregular procedure for health agencies.

The risk of bacterial contamination becomes imminent when beauty professionals are unaware of and do not adhere to biosafety measures, such as the use of personal protective equipment (PPE), disposal of single-use materials and hand hygiene procedures. Lack of knowledge about biosafety and how to conduct aesthetic procedures increases the risk of transmitting microorganisms to the professionals and patients who undergo the procedures. One of the characteristics of aesthetic work is direct contact with the patient. Beauty establishments are indulgent to the transmission of bacteria, whether by direct or indirect contact. This inability is the result of a lack of basic information about contamination and biosafety in beauty establishments.

Body piercing procedures are techniques that have been perfected over time and human culture, and nowadays practice invasive processes with piercing equipment or cutting materials, known as serious health risks if not handled correctly. The increase in people's interest in body piercing and the emergence of professionals in the field has benefited the techniques and establishments where the services take place. Professionals providing body piercing services can be important means of transmitting infectious microorganisms in the epidemiological chain, as they practice such activities at the limits of biosafety. However, users may not be properly informed about the risks of inadequate safety techniques, both in the establishment and in body piercing practices.

Transmission can happen through a small volume of blood resulting from visible or non-visible injuries between professionals and clients. There are many microorganisms that can be transmitted and spread by beauty services, including the skin and mucous membranes with abrasions and wounds. The recommendations for beauty professionals follow basic biosafety rules such as washing hands, wearing gloves, masks, goggles, aprons, disposing of contaminated material, and care must be taken when there is a risk or not, such as in the presence of blood, secretions and excretions from the skin and mucous membranes.

The risk of transmission to healthcare workers depends on the cause and prevalence of the illness, the patient's clinical circumstances, the presence and quantity of blood, the size of the bruise and the appropriate treatment after exposure. The most common and recurrent or simple bruises are percutaneous, caused by needles or other sharp objects. Mucocutaneous contusions are caused by droplets of blood or bodily fluids coming into contact with the eyes, nose, mouth or wounds that are already present, or by blood or fluids coming into contact with unharmed skin.

Nowadays, beautification techniques have spread among different social classes, ages and genders. However, the risks present in these practices must be observed, as they can cause serious damage to the health of professionals and clients. During these procedures, invasive practices are carried out on the skin, causing bleeding that favours infection by pathogenic microorganisms. The materials and equipment used can become vehicles for contaminating factors if they are not discarded or sterilised. Beautification activities that do not observe biosafety standards and do not practise decontamination and sterilisation procedures can cause bacterial infections and diseases, as well as dermatological lesions.

Although beauty and aesthetics establishments provide care, there are few records of contamination associated with professionals and patients, not because of the lack of occurrences, but because of the lack of notification, national and/or international epidemiological research, directed at and with an academic impact on this type of activity. The practical way in which beauty and aesthetics professionals work, due to a lack of qualification and discernment about biosafety recommendations, makes it necessary to discuss the risks of infection by microorganisms to professionals and to clients who adhere to aesthetic procedures.

The place where health professionals work doesn't always have the essential safety utensils needed to carry out procedures, such as gloves, aprons, masks, caps and goggles. In addition to the lack of materials, there are dysfunctions such as the absence of sinks for hand asepsis, alcohol gel, a container suitable for disposing of sharp objects, among others. These structures are indispensable for enabling professionals in the area to comply with biosafety methods. Correct hand cleaning is the most important tool for preventing and controlling infections in healthcare establishments, being the most relevant and least expensive. However, many professionals practice it unsatisfactorily, without considering the recommendations, and thus fail to carry out hand asepsis, which is inexcusable and extremely important, around 60% of the time. This criterion has thus been a major challenge due to the low adherence of health professionals to hand hygiene.

The epidermis manifests the greatest resistance to invasion by microorganisms, such as lesions caused by punctures, burns, scarifications, wounds or traumas that facilitate microbial penetration. Consequently, invasive techniques provide an access route for microbial transmission, so understanding and manipulating practices to destroy, remove or exclude infectious microorganisms is important for carrying out activities aimed at spreading diseases. Each pathology has its own method of control.

Micro-organisms are subdivided and identified into pathogenic and non-pathogenic, determined by whether they can cause disease. However, this distinction is not entirely satisfactory, as some micro-organisms are traditionally identified as non-pathogenic and therefore capable of causing disease.

In order to carry out professional beautification practices, it is recommended that you wear procedure gloves, goggles and masks. Gloves should be worn during contact with the user and the client. They should also be worn when decontaminating material and preparing for sterilisation. Protective goggles must be worn when decontaminating materials, and biosafety procedures help to avoid contact between solutions and the ocular mucosa, thus avoiding the risk of transmission by blood, fluids and secretions. The three pieces of personal protective equipment are of great importance in the process of degerming and decontaminating materials. Personal protective equipment is defined as gloves for each practice, an impenetrable apron, a cap, a mask and goggles, all of which are recommended to prevent health and safety at work.

Health professionals are exposed to various risks of accidents in the course of their work, and a hazard is considered to be a situation where there is the potential to cause harm. Biological risks are one of the most common during the course of their work. This corresponds to handling materials contaminated with blood and secretions.

Decontamination is the first stage in the procedure for sanitising utensils. This method involves washing the materials with soap and water, rinsing with running water and drying the materials used, after which they are sterilised. The glove is a favourable barrier to prevent the dermis from being exposed to pathogens that may be on the objects used in the practice. It also prevents direct contact with cleaning solutions, which can cause allergic processes. Disposable masks should be used both when attending to clients/patients and when avoiding direct contact with the sputum released by clients when talking or coughing. Protective goggles for individual use are recommended when handling blood, secretions and fluids.

The definition of safety is based on the assumption that every client can be contaminated with a pathogen and for this reason, professionals must use preventive measures whenever there is a likelihood of contact with blood or body fluids. The association of infection assessment is universally applied as a way of reducing occupational risks. All healthcare professionals need to use personal protective equipment frequently, such as barriers to protect against contact with blood and bodily fluids. The frequency and time of exposure of professionals to biological samples influences the risk of infection by pathogens. Environmental causes include increased contact with contaminated needles and sharp materials. An injury with a sharp object or needles is considered extremely serious and is capable of transmitting many pathogens.

Micro-organisms are most abundant under and around the fingernails on the hands, which are essential to our activities, and a large number of micro-organisms adhere to them when we touch objects. They can be transmitted to other people or to ourselves. Hand washing has become the main method of blocking contamination by micro-organisms and is always recommended, even when wearing gloves. Wash your hands before and after using disposable gloves, wear gloves continuously when working, replace them as soon as necessary and do not reuse them. Hands should always be washed after removing gloves, as the glove prevents contamination, but the glove's microporosity, vulnerability and removal can lead to hand contamination.

In order to assess contamination in healthcare facilities, it is essential to identify the types of objects used in various basic or specialised practices in the services provided to clients, and the materials must be listed according to their direct or indirect use. Instruments and materials soiled with biological samples such as blood, body fluids, secretions and excretions must be handled in such a way as to prevent contamination of the skin and mucous membranes, clothing and the transmission of microorganisms to other patients and environments. When cleaning, transferring or disposing of these objects, care must be taken to avoid accidents. They must be disposed of in suitable, rigid and impenetrable boxes, and the box must be closed when it reaches the permitted capacity, disposed of in a white contaminating rubbish bag for collection, and a needle must never be recapped after use.

Inert surfaces are conducive to the accumulation of pathogens and are not specifically correlated with the transmission of infection, but cleaning these surfaces is an active self-control in paralysing the epidemiological chain of contamination. It is important to carry out routine cleaning and decontamination of surfaces in the area and of equipment, even in places with simple physical structures. The workplace comprises the floor, walls, ceiling and doors, and the building contains chairs, tables, stretchers, benches, sinks, electronic equipment and materials exclusively for the care of each case.

Recent information requires objects and equipment to be cleaned to remove waste from the surface using automated or manual activities, physical (temperature) and chemical (detergents) with the use of water and detergents, after rinsing and drying. Before cleaning the material, it is important to wear PPE during the process. Decontamination is understood to be the procedure for destroying microorganisms (non-sporulated), fungi, viruses and protozoa, while disinfection is a procedure that does not destroy bacterial spores present on inanimate materials using physical or chemical means, based on the level of action.

Sterilisation is used for the complete removal of micro-organisms, where they can no longer be detected, including all proportions of them, including sporulated bacteria, and can even prevent infection and contamination. For sterilisation practices, a sterility protection level known as SAL (Sterility **Assurance Level**) of 10^{-6}, is determined, which is classified as a margin of prevention in sterilisation practices and is considered sterile when the viability of microorganisms is less than 1:1,000,000.

The autoclave is a piece of equipment used for sterilisation by moist heat. The biocidal operation is carried out by passing the latent heat from the steam to the materials, thus coagulating cell proteins and inactivating pathogenic microorganisms. The type of equipment used can be gravitational, from 132° to 135°, for a display period of 10 to 25 minutes; from 121° to 123°, for a display period of 15 to 30 minutes; pre-vacuum from 132° to 135°, for a display period of 3 to 4 minutes. Materials wrapped in paper of various types and objects wrapped in cloth must not come into contact with each other as they retain moisture. The object must be placed in such a way as to allow vapour to pass through, so that it is placed on the shelf in a vertical direction, utensil on utensil on the same shelf. The volumes must not come close to the walls of the chamber, and the weight must not reach 70 per cent of the internal capacity.

The storage and distribution of sterile materials, in terms of shelf life, varies depending on the type of coating, the effectiveness of the packaging, the storage environment in terms of humidity, and whether they are located on open or closed shelves, which will indicate the circulation of dust. However, for greater prevention, it is advisable to store packets in closed cabinets or crates for greater security. The opening of each sterilised packet and box should be done with septic procedures using sterile gloves or sterile tweezers specific to the practice. The circumstances of packaging and storage are relevant, making sure that all cleaning techniques are valid.

Sterilisation practices follow in the next steps:

1.   Steam inlet, Air outlet

2.   Sterilisation

3.   Drying

4.   Separate air access for internal pressure recovery

The apparatus has different ways of planning the steps, the exposure period and the use of distilled water, so each manufacturer's information must be followed.

Dry heat sterilisation uses the Pasteur oven, routinely known as an oven. Sterilisation is produced by heating and irradiating the heat, as it is less penetrable than moist heat. Dry heat is produced by resistors and is equipped with a thermostat, contact, resistor, pilot lamp, thermometer and switch. They require a longer period of exposure and greater heating. Objects that can be disinfected in an oven need to be heat-resistant, such as surgical equipment, stainless steel in general, ointments (as long as they are not damaged by the heat). The purpose of dry heat sterilisation is to eliminate micro-organisms by oxidation and cellular desiccation, so that the micro-organisms are denatured and die.

Heating should be monitored according to the type of object and individual validity.

•   *Chemical procedures:* glutaraldehyde, formaldehyde, peracetic acid, are suitable for delicate and thermosensitive utensils, which do not persist at the high temperatures of physical sterilisation practices.

•   *Physical procedures:* sterilisation using techniques can be carried out by by means of wet callus/autoclave, dry heat/greenhouse, or radiation/gamma rays/cobalt.

•   *Physical-chemical procedures:* ethylene oxide, peroxide plasma hydrogen, formaldehyde temperature.

In terms of physical sterilisation practices, the equipment most used by professionals and body piercers, due to its suitability and prevention, is the moist heat autoclave and the dry heat oven.

•   *Decontamination at a high level: this* is the complete elimination of vegetative forms of microorganisms, including *Mycobacterium tuberculosis,* viruses, fungi, and part of the spores, with the restriction of bacterial spores. It is suitable for semi-critical materials: the chemicals used are sodium hypochlorite, peracetic acid 02%, glutaraldehyde 02%.

•   *Decontamination at a medium level:* the technique paralyses the tubercle bacillus, bacteria in vegetative form, and most viruses, fungi, less bacterial spores, it is suitable for non-critical material that will come into contact with the epidermis, the chemical products used are chlorine-based compounds, phenolics and alcohols.

•   *Decontamination at a reduced level: the* procedure kills most bacteria, some viruses, fungi, does not eliminate resistant microorganisms such as tubercle bacillus and bacterial spores, and is suitable for non-critical materials.

•   *Critical materials:* penetrate the dermis and mucous membranes, enter the vascular system and subepithelial tissues, neutralise personal microbiota, and introduce objects to direct contact with blood or other infectious fluids. All of these phases that contain this procedure must be sterilised, materials such as:

surgical instruments, syringes, utensils that touch the dermis and mucosa are also considered critical.

• *Semi-critical materials:* they have contact with the dermis and mucous membranes and are therefore prepared to prevent the entry of subepithelial tissues, but to ensure their widespread use they need to undergo a high-level decontamination or sterilisation process. In objects such as tips, nebulisers, etc.

• *Non-critical materials:* these are used externally by the patient, are only in contact with the skin as a whole and the handling practices of healthcare professionals, requiring an individual cleaning or decontamination process at a reduced level (if the patient has been exposed to a biological sample), such as thermometers, buttons on equipment handled by the professional, tables, tubs and so on.

Disinfection indicators are chemical and biological. The external chemical ones are only used to distinguish the change in colour. Wraps that have already been decontaminated do not validate the procedure. Biological indicators are used to assess the applicability of the practice of sterilising cellulose strips, culture media or other materials contaminated by bacterial spores such as *Bacillus subtilis*. After the cycle, the indicators are incubated; if the procedure was efficient, the *Bacillus* colonies will not evolve.

The collection of delicate waste generated in healthcare establishments is a serious problem, which is reflected in the increase in the rate of pathogenic diseases recorded. The potential for infection, inefficient handling and lack of practice pose a risk to the health of the community and the population. Solid waste is understood to consist of objects no longer used in procedures, or those originating in nature. Generally, waste is determined according to its origin and the risks it poses to humans and the environment. According to ANVISA RDC No. 306/04 and CONAMA Resolution No. 358/2005, all practices related to human or animal health care are classified as producers of solid health waste.

CHAPTER 10

The importance of skin asepsis during aesthetic processes

10

Asepsis is the process that prevents micro-organisms (all those that can harm human health) from coming into contact with certain environments, organisms and objects. Given this information, it is important that hygiene and cleanliness are always up to date in order to prevent possible infections. The environment in which work is carried out must be hygienic, well-maintained and free from pathological germs.

There are ways of ensuring that the environment, equipment and objects are in the right conditions for the work to be carried out in the best possible way. One of these means is biosafety, which acts in these cases, where the main objective is to maintain patient and professional protection and safety. And it is through infection control measures that effective prevention can be achieved.

In addition to the asepsis process that is carried out before the patient undergoes the aesthetic process, measures such as: use of the appropriate PPE (personal protective equipment); sterilisation of instruments; disinfection of equipment and the environment are essential means of reducing and preventing possible infections and diseases that may occur.

In aesthetic establishments, the aforementioned biosafety is a rigorous process that must be taken into account. Lack of knowledge and poor behaviour in aesthetic procedures increases the risk of microorganisms being transmitted to the professionals and patients who undergo the procedures.

Beauty salons, dental practices and tattoo parlours are the main establishments where contamination by microorganisms is most prevalent, as they are characterised by direct contact with the patient.

Establishments must therefore follow the rules to guarantee the biosafety of the premises and prevent contamination. They must be strictly compliant with current health legislation. To this end, the recommendations for beauty professionals go hand in hand with the basic rules, such as washing hands, wearing gloves, caps, masks, goggles and aprons. In addition, the premises must have a rubbish bin with a plastic bag to dispose of contaminated waste. The internal structure should have smooth walls that make it easy to clean, remove debris, etc. These actions are essential to avoid the accumulation of microorganisms and dust.

Human skin is made up of three layers: epidermis, dermis and hypodermis. The asepsis process is necessary for better preparation when it comes to the aesthetic process, which involves techniques consisting of sharp objects, possible injuries during the process, among others. The skin is an important barrier for the introduction of exogenous substances and is characterised by the fact that it presents a pathway for the conduction of functional active ingredients.

Skin cleansing is a procedure that aims to remove blackheads, pimples, dead skin cells and other impurities that contribute to less elastic, less healthy skin. This procedure should be carried out by trained professionals, depending on your skin type (normal, oily and dry).

Thorough sanitisation of the skin is essential to prevent contamination by infectious agents. On the lipid side, hygienisation helps to maintain lower sebum production and increase tissue oxygenation, facilitating perspiration and better lubrication of the skin, providing a better condition for the mantle that surrounds it.

The use of suitable cosmetic chemical substances, provided they are also used effectively, can produce greater skin cleansing effects. It is up to the professional to check which products are most effective according to the patient's skin type.

Improving the efficacy and topical penetrability of substances is of paramount importance in the progression and improvement of medicines and cosmetics. Introduction into the skin takes place via three routes: transcellular, intracellular and follicular. The intracellular route was considered the most important and exclusive route of introduction for substances to be applied topically.

There are some processes that can help to sanitise the skin, such as the suction extraction technique, which consists of using vacuum therapy by means of a suction cup to use maximum suction during the procedure and requires skin cleansing, exfoliation, toning and emolliency. This technique should not generate pain or cause any discomfort on the surface of the patient's skin.

It's important to note that once the skin has been sanitised, the next step is to prepare it for the procedure to be carried out, i.e. to remove dead skin cells and other impurities, avoiding any contamination that could occur during the techniques used in this process.

Mention should also be made of the new aesthetic techniques used on the skin. One of these techniques is microneedling, also known as Dermaroller due to its brand name, which is not so new, but has been gaining ground since 2006. The method is carried out by breaking up the stratum corneum, without causing irregularities in the epidermis. The equipment consists of a cylindrical roller coated with small, thin needles made of pure surgical steel or titanium alloy, with variable amplitude sizes.

Microneedling also creates microchannels causing collagen to be produced, which makes wound healing and skin conditioning more effective. As well as stimulating collagen production, microneedling has been used to facilitate the penetration of pharmacological cosmetics and growth factors, which are biologically active substances. Most of these factors have huge hydrophilic molecules, preventing them from penetrating the epidermis in quantities that can be measured to produce beneficial effects.

The microneedling technique is a highly effective way of treating acne blemishes. These, in turn, are caused by acne, which mainly affects the face. Acne spots and scars act on the facial skin, which from the outset is a challenge to treat and remove. There are various techniques, such as chemical peels. But most of these treatment techniques are ineffective or don't produce satisfactory results. In view of these techniques, the risks of contamination associated with the products must be analysed, observing the need for their use.

CHAPTER 11

Biotechnological analysis in microbiology

Microorganisms are part of nature's cycles and are responsible for the balance of ecosystems and are fundamental in food chains. However, only 10% of the microorganisms that exist on the planet have been characterised and described. This means that only 1% of the planet's bacteria and viruses are known, and only 5% of fungi.

Molecular biology works as a great aid in differentiating species through molecular evaluation. Every day, more species of bacteria are discovered on the planet. They are differentiated through their genes or genetic material, and it is estimated that there are around 20,000 to 40,000 bacterial species.

It is estimated that less than 1% of the bacteria in the biosphere are known to exist. They are bacteria with highly specialised characteristics capable of withstanding high temperatures, salt concentrations and extreme pH values. They are unusual metabolisers such as sulphate reducers and methanogens.

The new techniques have highlighted the enormous genetic diversity of bacteria present in just one gram of soil. Given that around 5,000 species of bacteria have been described, most of which are not from soils, there is a huge knowledge gap to be filled in biodiversity studies.

It is estimated that only 5 per cent of existing fungi have been described. Progress has been made in cataloguing macroscopic fungi (mushrooms), which have many studies.

The aim of molecular methods for identifying fungi is to understand evolutionary relationships and their characteristics and mechanisms.

The vast majority of fungi contribute to the evolution of life, are biologically present microorganisms, with pathogenic species, and are also little known, as approximately 0.5 per cent of the fungal population has been identified.

Viruses are very small infectious agents with no cellular structure, containing only one type of nucleic acid. Viruses are obligate intracellular parasites, and through molecular techniques they are characterised and identified.

The combination of molecular biology and bioinformatics has not only helped to discover and characterise species, but also to store their data in databases so that it can be analysed as patterns and compared to other primitive sequences. This helps to discover new species.

It is important to emphasise that a large part of the advances associated with modern biotechnology and agriculture are derived from recent discoveries in the fields of genetics, physiology, molecular biology, bioinformatics and the metabolism of microorganisms.

THE DERMARROLLER

Microneedling has recently gained greater visibility in the medical and aesthetic fields. Demand for these techniques has increased by around 43 per cent. This treatment makes multiple perforations in the epidermis without serious damage, stimulating collagen and thickening the skin.

The device used in the treatment "is a drum-shaped roller studded with 192 fine micro-needles in eight rows, 0.5 - 1.5 mm long and 0.1 mm in diameter. The equipment is pre-sterilised and, depending on the manufacturer, the number of needles can vary up to 540, as can their length, which can range from 0.25mm to 3.0mm.

Before starting treatment, the area where the equipment and instruments will be used should be sanitised with 70% alcohol. A topical anaesthetic should be applied before treatment. The tool is rolled over the desired area vertically, horizontally and diagonally right and left, 10 to 15 times in each direction, causing an average of 250 - 300 micropunctures/cm^2 Only 70% of the length of the needle penetrates the epidermis. After treatment, the skin is hyperemic, sensitive and oedematous, and remains so for a maximum of 3 days. Topical vitamins such as A and E are needed to help stimulate collagen.

When the needlestick injury occurs, an inflammatory healing process begins, which has three phases: injury, healing and maturation. Five days after the injury, the fibronectin matrix is formed, allowing collagen to be deposited just below the basal layer of the epidermis. Due to this injury and the inflammatory response, it is estimated that microneedling is effective in the aesthetic treatment of acne scars.

This technique is contraindicated in cases of predisposition to keloid formation, diabetes, neuromuscular disease, haemorrhagic disorder, collagen disease, acute or chronic corticosteroids, anticoagulant treatment, the presence of skin cancer, warts, solar keratoses or any skin infection and pregnancy.

In order to minimise the impact of these problems on the aesthetics market, it is advisable to adopt standard measures used in healthcare environments around the world, which we call biosafety.

Biological risks include viruses, bacteria, parasites, protozoa, fungi and bacilli. These risks occur through direct contact with the individual, the environment or any contaminated material. The main ones are bacteria, which need a mode of transport for their proliferation in the environment. These are: hands, clothing, equipment, utensils and contact surfaces, also due to the formation of biofilm.

BACTERIA PRESENT IN THE SKIN'S MICROBIOTA

Biological contamination occurs cutaneously or percutaneously, with or without lesions, airborne (respiratory), conjunctival (skin), oral (ingestion) and ocular (conjunctival mucosa). There are various bacteria resident in the normal microbiota, including **Staphyloccocus sp** and **Escherichia coli.** As this is an invasive method and the equipment is often reused, the microorganism can penetrate and cause an infection.

The genus **Staphylococcus** is made up of spherical bacteria known to be grouped together in grape clusters. **Staphylococcus aureus,** even though it is part of the normal microbiota of the skin, is considered to be a species of bacteria responsible for causing a wide range of bacterial infections of concern to human health, and today it is a bacterium that has acquired a wide capacity for resistance to some antimicrobials.

Staphylococcus aureus is a Gram-positive bacterium that can cause infections by breaking down the skin barrier. The tissue is the area of greatest domination, with an average prevalence of 40% in the adult population. The aforementioned bacteria do not pose a risk and are able to survive for a while without harming human health. These microorganisms are associated with inflammation of the skin and soft tissues, and are capable of causing more serious and fatal illnesses.

This bacterial species has the ability to cause long-term inflammation and can increase in cases of pathological skin manifestations with chronic infections. Skin infections such as topical dermatitis, psoriasis and acne, among others, have been linked to a disturbance in the normal microbiota of the skin, and the expansion of infectious microorganisms such as **Stapylococcus aureus** has been reported as a potent device for skin inflammation, aiding in long-term skin infection by promoting the colonisation of bacteria.

Staphylococcus epidermidis inhabits various areas of the epidermis and is classified as a commensal, but can also operate as an opportunistic pathogen in which it invades the skin surface and enters the bloodstream. The comparison of the genome and the distinction of **Staphylococcus epidermidis** identified genetic elements with characteristics for many considerable functions and antibiotic resistance involving bactericins such as epidermin, an isolate with antimicrobial action.

Staphylococcus epidermidis live as infectious microorganisms when they invade an open lesion, the precision of microbiota treatment increases the selectivity of the fermentation activities of **Staphylococcus epidermidis** against acne. The increase in sucrose as an intercession is conducted specifically for the fermentation of **S. epidermidis,** and can be relatively safe when used to balance acne.

Streptococci are facultative anaerobic bacteria that grow predominantly in atmospheric air. The evolution of the species is driven by an increase in carbon dioxide (CO_2). **Streptococci** characteristically develop in chains (diplococci) when growing in broth media. Since the pathogens have several features that aid their virulence, the human skin and mucosa are the only reservoirs for group A **streptococcus** bacteria. **Streptococcus Pyogenes** is a group A **streptococcus** (GAS) and can be responsible for causing infections of varying degrees, from mild infections such as pharyngitis and impetigo to serious infections such as necrotising fasciitis and streptococcal toxic shock syndrome.

To diagnose beta haemolytic **streptococcus** colonies, the biological material collected is sown in a petri dish containing blood agar culture medium, using antiseptic procedures and incubating for 24 hours in a bacteriological oven, then using the catalase technique, where the result is usually positive, visualising its morphology microscopically.

Escherichia coli is a prevalent species in the human microbiota and is associated with poor hygiene on the part of handlers. It belongs to the **Enterobacteriaceae** family and is a Gram-negative rod. Proliferative at temperatures between 7°C and 48°C, catalase positive, oxidase negative, ph close to neutral, a species prevalent in the human microbiota. It is among the microorganisms that cause infections.

Escherichia coli present in water and food is a strong denomination of contamination. Faecal bacteria are classified as a storehouse of potential antimicrobial resistance genes, and can transfer these genes to the bacteria of origin when conducted in transferable or mobile genetic elements, this flow of resistant genes establishes a danger to human health.

METHODOLOGIES USED TO ANALYSE MICROORGANISMS IN THE DERMAROLLER

Microbiological analyses can be carried out using a variety of techniques. The correct confirmation of the diagnosis is prepared by isolating and identifying bacteria using samples taken at the site of infection, practices known as bacteriological examinations or culture. There are also other techniques that can be used to diagnose microorganisms. Means that use procedures to confirm infectious agents directly from collected clinical material are of great interest because they are quick and do not require cultivation techniques.

The first step in the process of clinical sampling for identification is the microscopic analysis of the material collected. Direct examination is agile and inexpensive, the study of microorganisms can point to aetiological agents and guides the professional in choosing the most suitable cultures for obtaining results. Cell and microorganism samples are often translucent and can be distinguished using dyes. Direct observation of biological material fixed between slides and coverslips provides information on the cellular composition, morphology and motility of the infectious agent. Microbiological identification of bacterial virulence takes place through isolation and phenotypic and biochemical definition, which in some cases are time-consuming, expensive and sometimes unfeasible techniques.

The risks of contamination associated with products must be analysed in the light of the need for their use. Microbial transmission is a problem that influences both customer self-confidence and the quality of the product, equipment and so on. It is necessary to ensure that the microbial load is probably lower than legally permitted, as well as the absence of pathogenic microorganisms.

There are other methods, such as washing the equipment in saline, plating and then observing the colony for biochemical characterisation. This procedure can also be carried out using a Drigalsky loop.

These microbiological methods should be carried out as quality control of the equipment to prevent infections and help with the quality of aesthetic procedures.

Employees

Chapter AUTHORS

Chapter 01 - Paulo Sérgio da paz Silva Filho

Chapter 02 - Imayra Zuilla Cardoso Silva

Chapter 03 - Hernande Pereira Passos Júnior

Chapter 04 - Joina Meneses de Oliveira

Chapter 05 - Mariana lopes da silva

Chapter 06 - Jadielson da Silva Santos

Chapter 07 - Francisca Faustilene da Silva Ribeiro

Chapter 08 - Ana Caroline Ribeiro de Miranda

Chapter 09 - Valdir Morais Silva Júnior

Chapter 10 - Jucyara do nascimento rodrigues

Chapter 11 - Kelly Maria Rêgo da Silva

References

ALARCÓN, O.C.; ORDENES, P.M.C.; DENEGRI, M.M.; ZÚNIGA, J. Infecciones invasoras por Streptococcus bhemolítico Grupo A.Revista chilena de pediatría, v.77, n.5, p.487-491, 2006.

ALBERTINI, B.B.; SOUZA, F.G.L.; Action of microneedling on people with acne scars.

ALETHEA, TRICIA - **Microneedling part II**- Revista NegócioEstética, 2013. ALMEIDA, G.C.M. et al. Nasal colonisation by Staphylococcussp. in hospitalised patients. Acta Paul Enferm, v.27, n.3,p.273-9, 2014.

ALTUN, O. et al. Rapid Identification of Microorganisms from Sterile Body Fluids by Use of FilmArray. **Journal of Clinical Microbiology**, v.53, n.2, p.710-712, 2015.

AN, B.; LIN, Y-S.; BRODSKY, B. Collagen interactions: Drug design and deliver. **Advanced Drug Delivery Reviews**, 2016; 97: 69-84.

ANDRÉ.L.SANTOS, et al; Staphylococcus aureus: visiting a strain of hospital importance. **J. Brasil. Patol. Med. Lab**. V.34,n.6, p.413-423, 2007.

ASIF, M.; KANODIA, S.; SINGH, K. Combined autologous platelet-rich plasma with microneedling verses microneedling with distilled water in the treatment of atrophic acne scars: a concurrent split-face study. **Journal of Cosmetic Dermatology**, v.15, p.434-443, 2016.

AUST, M.C.; FERNANDES, D.; KOLOKYTHAS, P.; KAPLAN, H.M.; VOGT, P.M. Percutaneous collagen induction therapy: An alternative treatment for scars, wrinkles and skin laxity. **Plast Reconstr Surg**, 21:1421-9, 2008.

AUST, M.C.; REIMERS, K.; HAPLAN, H.M.; STAHL, F.; REPENNING, C.; SCHEPER, T.; JAHN, S.; SCHEAIGER, N.; IPAKTCHI, R.; REDEKER, J.;

ALTINTAS, M.A.; VOGT, P.M. Percutaneous collagen induction - regeneration in place of cicatrisation? **Journal of Plastic, Reconstructive & Aesthetic Surgery**, 64, 97-107, 2011.

BHATNAGAR, S.; DAVE, K.; VENUGANTI, V. V. K. Microneedles in the clinic. **Journal of Controlled Release**, v. 260, p. 164-182, 2017.

BIASOLI, A. M. Acne. **In:** Shirlei Borelli. Oleg (Orgs). **Cosmiatry in Dermatology**. São Paulo: Roca, 2007.

BORGHETI[1] , S.P. VIEGAS[2] , K. CAREGNATO[3] , R. C. A. Biosecurity **in central sterile services department: the doubts of professionals; Bioseguridad em El centro de materiales y esterelizacion: dudas de lós profesionales. Rev. Sobecc, São Paulo. Jan/Mar. 2016; 21 (1): 3-12.**

BRANDT, H.R.C.; ARNONE, M.; VALENTE, N.Y.S; CRIADO, P.R.; SOTTO, M.N.; Cutaneous small vessel vasculitis: aetiology, pathogenesis, classification and diagnostic criteria - Part I *, **Anais Brasileiros de Dermatologia**, v.82, n.5, p.387-406, 2007

BULL, A. T.; MARRS, B.L. & KURANE, R.. Biotechnology for clean industrial products and processes. p. 1-200. *In:* Towards industrial sustainability. **Organisation for Economic Cooperation and Development**, Paris. 1998.

BULL, A. T.; WARD, A. C. & GOODFELLOW, M.. Search and discovery strategies for biotechnology:the paradigm shift. **Microbiology and Molecular Biology Reviews**, 64(3): 573-606. 2000.

CAMIRAND, A.; DOUCET, J. Needle dermabrasion. **J Cutan Aesthet Surg**, 21:48-51,1997.

CAMPOS, A.C.L.; BORGES-BRANCO, A.; GROTH, A.K.; Wound healing. Arquivos Brasileiros de Cirurgia Digestiva. v.20, n.1, p.51-58, 2007.

CANAL, N. et al. Characterisation oh the variable region in the class 1 integron of antimicrobial - resisant Escherichia coli isolated from surface water. **Brazilian Journal of Microbiology,** v.47, n.2, p.337-344.

CANCELLARA, A.D. et al. Multicentric study of invasive infections by Streptococcus pyogenes in Argentina.Arch. Argent. Pediatr, v.114, n.3, p.199- 207, 2016.

CANHOS, V. P.; MANFIO, G. P. **Microbiological Resources for Biotechnology Canhos & Manfio.** Microbiological Resources for Biotechnology. Available at:< http://www.mct.gov.br/upd blob/0000/439.pdf>. Accessed on: 05 July 2017. CANSINO, N.D.S.C. et al. Effect of ultrasound on survival and growth of Escherichia coli in cactus pear juice during storage. **Brazilian Journal of Microbiology,** v.47, n.2, p.431-437, 2016.

CHALKER, V.J. et al. Integration of Genomic and Other Epidemiologic Data to Investigate and Control a Cross-Institutional Outbreak of Streptococcus pyogenes. Emerg. Infect. Dis., v.22, n.6, p.973-980, 2016.

CHAWLA, S. Split Face Comparative Study of Microneedling with PRP Versus Microneedling with Vitamin C in Treating Atrophic Post Acne Sears. **Journal of Cutaneous and Aesthetic Surgery**, v.7, n.4, p.209-212, 2014.

CHAWLA, S. Split Face Comparative Study of Microneedling with PRP Versus Microneedling with Vitamin C in Treating Atrophic Post Acne Scars. **Journal of Cutaneous and Aesthetic Surgery**, v.7, n.4, p.209-212, 2014.

CHRISTENSEN, G.J.M. et al. Antagonism Between Staphylococcus Epidermidis and Propionibacterium Acnes and its Genomic Basis. **BioMed Central - BMC,** v.17, n.152, p.1-14,2016.

CHUNG, H. J.; UITTO, J. Type VII Collagen: The Anchoring Fibril Protein at Fault in Dystrophic Epidermolysis Bullosa. **Dermatologic Clinics,** 2010; 28(1): 93-105 COLWELL, R. Microbial diversity: the importance of exploration and conservation. **Journal of Industrial Microbiology and Biotechnology,** 18:5, 302-307.

COSTA[1] ,L.P. et al,. Accidentes **de trabajo com enfermeros de** clínica médica **involucrando material** biológico; **Accidents with biological material involving clinical medicine nurses.** 2015.16544

CUNHA, M.G; PARAVIC, F.D; MACHADO, C.A. Histological changes in collagen types after different treatment modalities for dermal remodelling: a literature review. **Surgical And Cosmetic Dermatology,** v.7, n.4, p.285-92, 2015.

DA SILVA, T. F., & PENNA, A. L. B. Collagen: Chemical characteristics and functional properties. **Journal of the Adolfo Lutz Institute,** v. 71, n. 3, p. 530-539, 2012.

DALBONE, NAWAHLE et al - Microneedling as an agent that enhances the permeation of body active ingredients in the treatment of localised lipodystrophy - VIII EPCC - Encontro internacional de Produção Cientifica Cesumar, October 2014. DINIZ, A.F.; MATTÉ, G.R. Biosafety procedures adopted by beauty service professionals. **Biosafety procedures adoptedbybeautyprofessional,** v.22, n.3, p.751-759, 2013.

DINIZ, A.F.; MATTÉ, G.R. Biosafety procedures adopted by beauty professionals. **Biosafety procedures adopted by beauty professionals,** v.22, n.3, p.751-759, 2013.

DINIZ, A.F.; MATTÉ, G.R. Biosafety procedures adopted by beauty professionals. **Biosafety procedures adopted by beauty professionals,** v.22, n.3, p.751-759, 2013.

DODDABALLAPUR, S. Microneedling with Dermaroller. **J Cutan Aesthet Surg,** Jul-Dec;2(2): 110-111, 2009.

DODDABALLAPUR, S. Microneedling with dermaroller. **Journal Of Cutaneous And Aesthetic Surgery,** Bangalore, Karnataka, India, v. 2, n. 2, p. 110-111, 2009.

DODDABALLAPUR, S. Microneedling with dermaroller. **Journal Of Cutaneous And Aesthetic Surgery,** Bangalore, Karnataka, India, v. 2, n. 2, p. 110-111, Jul./Dec. 2009. DODDABALLAPUR, Satish. Microneedling with dermaroller. **Journal of cutaneous and aesthetic surgery,** v. 2, n. 2, p. 110, 2009.

DODDABALLAPUR, Satish. Microneedlingwithdermaroller. Journalofcutaneousandaestheticsurgery, v. 2, n. 2, p. 110, 2009.

DONATELLI[1] , S. et al,. Accidents **with biological material:** an **approach based on the analysis of** work activities. Saúde soc. Vol.24 no.4 são Paulo oct./Dec.2015

DRAELOS, Z. D. **Procedures in cosmetic dermatology:** Cosmeceuticals. 1 ed.Rio de Janeiro: Elsevier, 2005.

EL-DOMYATI, Moetaz et al. Microneedlingtherapy for atrophic acne scars: anobjectiveevaluation. The

Journal of clinical and aesthetic dermatology, v. 8, n. 7, p. 36, 2015.

EVANGELISTA, S.S.; OLIVEIRA, A.C. Community-acquired methicillin-resistant *staphylococcus* **aureas**: a worldwide problem/ community-acquired methicillin-resistant *staphylococcus aureas*: a worldwide problem. **Revista Brasileira de Enfermagem,** v.68, n.1, 2015.

EVANGELISTA, S.S.; OLIVEIRA, A.C. *Staphylococcusaureasmeticilino* resistente adquirido na comunidade: um problema mundial/ *staphylococcus* **áureasmeticilino** - resistente adquirido em lacomunidad: um problema mundial. **Revista Brasileira de Enfermagem,** v.68, n.1, 2015.

FAUZI, M.B., et al. Ovine tendon collagen: Extraction, characterisation and fabrication of thinfilms for tissue engineering applications. **Materials Science and Engineering C**, 2016; 68:163-171

FEITOSA, G.P.V.; OLIVEIRA, E.C.; HIGUCHI, C. T.; GOMES, J.P.C.; BARBOSA, I.T.F. **Critical analysis of microdermabrasion techniques by blasting and sanding: Literature Review.** InterfacEHS - Health, Environment and Sustainability Vol. 11 no 2 - December 2016, São Paulo: Senac University Centre.

FERREIRA, W.; ÁVILA, S. L. M. **Diagnóstico Laboratorial das Principais Doenças Infecciosas e Auto-Imunes.** São Paulo, Guanabara-Koogan, 2nd Edition, 2001.

FRAZEN, J; SANTOS, J; ZANCANARO, V. COLLAGEN: AN APPROACH TO AESTHETICS, **Caçador,** v.2, n.2, p. 49-61, 2013.

FUNÇÃO, J.M. NARCHI, N.Z. Research into Group B streptococcus in pregnant women in the East Zone of São Paulo, **Revista da Escola de Enfermagem da USP,** v.47, n.1, p.22- 29, 2013.

GARBACCIO JL, OLIVEIRA AC. Biosafety and occupational risk among beauty and aesthetics professionals: an integrative review. **Rev Eletronica Enferm.** 2012;14(3):702-11.

GARBACCIO, J. L.; OLIVEIRA, A. C. Hidden risk in the aesthetics and beauty segment: an evaluation of professionals' knowledge and biosafety practices in beauty salons. **Revista Texto e Contexto Enfermagem,** v.22, n.4, p.989-98, 2013.

GARBACCIO, J. L.; OLIVEIRA, A. C. Hidden risk in the aesthetics and beauty segment: an evaluation of professionals' knowledge and biosafety practices in beauty salons. **Revista Texto e Contexto Enfermagem,** v. 22, n. 4, p. 989-98, 2013.

GARBACCIO, J.L.; OLIVEIRA, A.C. Hidden risk in the aesthetics and beauty segment: an evaluation of professionals' knowledge and biosafety practices in beauty salons. **Revista Texto e Contexto Enfermagem,** v.22, n.4, p.989-98, 2013.

GARBACCIO, J.L.; OLIVEIRA, A.C. Hidden risk in the aesthetics and beauty segment: an evaluation of professionals' knowledge and biosafety practices in beauty salons. **Revista Texto e Contexto Enfermagem,** v.22, n.4, p.989-98, 2013.

GARBACCIO, J.L.; OLIVEIRA, A.C. Hidden risk in the aesthetics and beauty segment: an evaluation of professionals' knowledge and biosafety practices in beauty salons. **Revista Texto e Contexto Enfermagem,** v.22, n.4, p.989-98, 2013.

GARG, Shilpa; BAVEJA, Sukriti. Combinationtherapy in the management ofatrophic acne scars. Journal ofcutaneousandaestheticsurgery, v. 7, n. 1, p. 18, 2014.

group A hyper-virulence in the human pathogen LIMA, M.F.P.; BORGES, M.A.; PARENTE, R.S.; JÚNIOR, R.C.V.; OLIVEIRA, M.E. Staphylococcus aureus and Hospital Infections - Literature Review. RevistaUningá Review, v.21, n.1, p.32- 39, 2015.

HAMMOND. The current magnitude of biodiversity. In: **Global Biodiversity Assessment**. . 1997.

HARRIS, Adam G.; NAIDOO, Catherine; MURRELL, Dedee F. Skinneedling as a treatment for acne scarring: Anup-to-date reviewoftheliterature.

International Journal of Women's Dermatology, v. 1, n. 2, p. 77-81, 2015.

HARTMANN, D; RUZICKA, T.; GAUGLITZ, G.G. Complications associated with cutaneous aesthetic procedures. **J Dtsch Dermatol Ges**, v. 13, n. 8, p. 778-786, 2015. HELENA FAGUNDES; CARLOSA.F.O et al; Inflammatory Infections Caused by Staphylococcus aureus and their Implications for Public Health. **Ciência Rual**, v.34, n.4, p. 1315-1320,2004.

HUGENHOLTZ, P. & PACE, N.R. Identifying microbial diversity in the natural environment: a molecular phylogenetic approach. **Trends in Biotechnology**, 14: 190197. . 1996.

HUGENHOLTZ, P.; GOEBEL, B. M. & PACE, N. R. Impact of culture-independent studies on the emerging phylogenetic view of bacterial diversity. **J. Bacteriology**, 180: 4765-4774. 1998.

HUGENHOLTZ, P.; PITULLE, C.; HERSHBERGER, K. L. & PACE, N.R. b. Novel division-level bacterial diversity in a Yellowstone hot spring. **J. Bacteriology**, 180: 366-376. 1998.

HUNTER-CEVERA,. **The value of microbial diversity.** Current Opinion in Microbiology 1: 278-285. 1998.

ISIHI, C.M.A. **Evaluation of biosafety conditions and risk perception of tattooists and body piercers in relation to hepatitis B and C virus infection in the city of São Paulo.** Dissertation. Disease Control Coordination of the São Paulo State Health Department. São Paulo. 2010. 147f.

ISIHI, C.M.A. **Evaluation of biosafety conditions and risk perception of tattooists and body piercers in relation to hepatitis B and C virus infection in the city of São Paulo.** Dissertation. Disease Control Coordination of the São Paulo State Health Department. São Paulo. 2010. 147f. JACKELINE G. da Silva, et al; antimicrobial activity of the extract of AnacardiumOccidentaleLinn. on multidrug-resistant samples of staphylococcusaureus.**Revista Brasileira. Farmacognosia,**v.17, n.4, p. 572-577,2007. KALIL, C.L.P.V. Treatment of acne scars with the microneedling and drug delivery technique. **Surgical Cosmetic Dermatology,** v.7, n.2. p.144-8, 2015.

KALIL, C.L.P.V.; FRAINER, R.H.; DEXHEIMER, L.S.; TONOLI, R.E.; BOFF, A.L. Treatment of acne scars using the microneedling and drug delivery technique. **Surgical & Cosmetic Dermatology**, p. 144.

KATE, K. & LAIRD, S. A. (eds.), The commercial use of biodiversity. Earthscan **Publications Ltd., London,** U.K. 1999.

KLAYN, A. P.; LIMANA, M. D.; MOARES, L. R. S. Microneedling as an agent that enhances the permeation of body active ingredients in the treatment of localised lipodystrophy: a case study. In: ENCONTRO INTERNACIONAL DE PRODUÇÃO CIENTÍFICA CESUMAR - EPCC, 8.p. 1-5, 2013, Maringá. **Electronic Proceedings**... Maringá: Editora Cesumar, 2013.

LEÃO, C.S. et al. Evaluation of cytokines produced by B-hemolytic streptococcus in acute praryagotonsillitis.**Brazilian Journal of Otorhinolaryngology**, v.81, n.4, p.402- 407, 2015.

LEÃO, C.S. et al. Evaluation of cytokines produced by B-hemolytic streptococcus in acute praryagotonsillitis. **Brazilian Journal of Otorhinolaryngology**, v.81, n.4, p.402- 407, 2015.

LEE, H. J. et al. Efficacy of microneedling plus human stem cell conditioned medium for skin rejuvenation: a randomized, controlled, blinded split-face study. **Annals of Dermatology**, v. 26, n. 5, p. 584-591, 2014.

LIMA, A. A.; SOUZA, T. H.; GRIGNOLI, L. C. E. The benefits of microneedling in the treatment of aesthetic dysfunctions. **Revista científica da FHO|UNIARARAS**, v.3, n.1, p.92-99, 2015.

LIMA, A.A.; SOUZA, T.H.; GRIGNOLI, L.C.E. The benefits of microneedling in the treatment of aesthetic dysfunctions. **Revista científica da FHO|UNIARARAS**, v.3, n.1, p.92-99, 2015.

LIMA, A.A.; SOUZA, T.H.; GRIGNOLI, L.C.E.; The benefits of microneedling in the treatment of aesthetic dysfunctions. Revista científica da FHO. v.3, n.1, 2015.

LIMA, E. A. Association of microneedling with phenol peeling: a new therapeutic proposal for sagging, wrinkles and acne scars on the face. **Surgical Cosmetic Dermatology**, v. 7, n. 4, 2015.

LIMA, E. V. A.; LIMA, M. A.; TAKANO, D. Microneedling: experimental study and classification of the injury caused. **Surgical & Cosmetic Dermatology**, Rio de Janeiro, v. 5, n. 2, p. 110-114, Apr./Jun. 2013.

LIMA, E.A. Association of microneedling with phenol peeling: a new therapeutic proposal for sagging, wrinkles and acne scars on the face. **Surgical Cosmetic Dermatology**, v.7, n.4, 2015.

LIMA[a] , E.V.A.; LIMA[b] , M.A.; TAKANO, D. Microneedling: experimental study and classification of the injury caused. **Surgical Cosmetic Dermatology**, v.5, n.2, p.110- 4, 2013.

LISA, R.; HENK, H.; ALI, P.; FILIP, S.; STAN, M. Microneedling: Where do we stand now? A systematic review of the literature. **Journal of Plastic, Reconstructive & Aesthetic Surgery**, p. 1-14, 2017.

LOPES, V.K. et al. Multidrug-resistant *Staphylococcusaureasinfections*: treatment and prophylaxis: treatmentandprophylaxis. **Brazilian Journal of Medicine,** v.102, n.4, p., 2014.

LOPES, V.K. et al. Multidrug - resistant **Staphylococcus** *aureas infections*: treatment and prophylaxis. **Brazilian Journal of Medicine**, v.102, n.4, p., 2014.

MACÁRIO, F.E.C. **Analysis of the resources used in the treatment of sagging skin by professional physiotherapists in Brazil.** 2014.

MAJID, I. Microneedling Therapy in Atrophic Facial Scars: An Objective Assessment. **J Cutan Aesthet Surg**, Jan-Jun; 2(1): 26-30, 2009.

MAJID, Imran. Microneedlingtherapy in atrophic facial scars: anobjectiveassessment. Journalofcutaneousandaestheticsurgery, v. 2, n. 1, p. 26, 2009.

MARTIGNAGO, C.C.S.; VILLANOVA, V.H.; REBONATO, T.A.; REMLINGER, R.; DEON, K. C. **Galvanic microcurrent as a physiotherapeutic resource for the treatment of stretch marks.** State University of the Centre-West of Paraná/Sector of Health Sciences, 2009.

MATOS, MARINA CRUZ DE OLIVEIRA. **The use of microneedling in the aesthetic treatment of acne scars.** Article presented to the Bachelor of Aesthetics course at IBMR - Laureate International Universities, as part of the requirements for obtaining the degree of Bachelor of Aesthetics. Rio de Janeiro. 2014.

MAUAD, R. **Estética e cirurigia plástica, tratamento no pré e pós operatório.** 2 ed. São Paulo: Senac, 2003.

MCCRUDDEN, M. T. C.; MCALISTER, E.; COURTENAY, A. J.; GONZATEZ- VA'ZQUEZ, P.; RAJ SINGH, T. R.; DONNELLY, R. F. Microneedle applications in improving skin appearance. **Exp Dermatol** v. 24, n. 8, p. 561-566, 2015.

MENEZES, C.R. et al. Effect of microwave radiation on the inactivation of **Escherichia Coli** strains. **Department of Food Science and Technology,** v.30, n.256-257, 2016.

MILLER, E.W. et al. Regulatory rewiring confers serotype-specific hyper-virulence in the human pathogen group A Streptococcus. Molecular Microbiology, v.98, n.3, p.473- 489, 2015.

MOREIRA A, BAMBACE J, OLAVO A, JORGE C. Efficacy of chlorexidine aqueous solutions to disinfect surfaces. **Rev Biociência.** 2003;9:73-81.

MUSSER, J.M. et al. Streptococcus pyogenes causing toxic-shock-like syndrome and other invasive diseases: Clonal diversity and pyrogenic exotoxin expression. Proc. Natl. Acad. Sci, v.88, p.2668-2672, 1991.

MYERS. Environmental services of biodiversity. Proc. **Natl. Acad. Sci.** USA, 93(7): 2764-2769. 1996.

NAIR, P. A.; ARORA, T. H. Microneedling using dermaroller a means of collagen induction therapy. **Gujarat Medical Journal.** v.69, n. 1, p 24-27, 2014.

NEGRÃO, Mariana C. P. Microneedling: physiological bases and practices. CR8 Editora, 2015.

NEVES, J.D.B.; VANDESMET V.C.S.; MENDES, C.F.C.; JÚNIOR, D.L.S.; SANTOS, N.M.; CORDEIRO, P.M.D.; LEANDRO, L.M.G. **Bacteriological analysis of lab coats worn by health professionals at a school clinic in the city of Juazeiro do Norte, Ceará.** Rev Interfaces [Internet] Vol. 3(9), pp. 50-54, 22 April, 2016

OLIVEIRA, L. S.; ROSSATO, L. G.; BERTOL, C. D. Analysis of the microbiological contamination of different dentifrices/ Microbiological contamination evaluation of different dentrifices. **Revista de Ondontologia da Unesp,** v.45, n.2, p.85-89, 2016. OLIVEIRA, L.S.; ROSSATO, L.G.; BERTOL, C.D. Análise da contaminação microbiológica de diferentes dentifrícios/ Microbiological contamination evaluation of different dentrifices. **Revista de Ondontologia da Unesp,** v.45, n.2, p.85-89, 2016.

OLIVEIRA, L.S.; ROSSATO, L.G.; BERTOL, C.D. Analysis of the microbiological contamination of different dentifrices/ Microbiological contamination evaluation of different dentrifices. **Revista de Ondontologia da Unesp,** v.45, n.2, p.85-89, 2016. OLIVEIRA, L.S.; ROSSATO, L.G.; BERTOL, C.D.

Análise da contaminação microbiológica de diferentes dentifrícios/ Microbiological contamination evaluation of different dentrifices. **Revista de Ondontologia da Unesp,** v.45, n.2, p.85-89, 2016.

PAGANI, B. B.; COSTA, L. V. M.; VALDAMERI, G. A. Skin hygiene with suction extraction - a demonstration of the technique and results.
University of Vale do Itajaí - UNIVALI, Florianópolis, Santa Catarina, 2005.

PATO, C.T.C. Streptococcuspyogenes as an agent of skin and soft tissue infection. Dissertation. University of Lisbon Faculty of Sciences - Department of Plant Biology. 2011. 37f.

PEDROSO, M.G.V. et al. **Comparative study of hydrolysed and commercial collagen with added PVA.** Dissertation. Chemistry Institute of São Carlos, University of São Paulo. 2009. 61f.

PEREIRA, B.B.; TERRUEL, D.D.S.; CARRILLO, M.F.B. **TREATMENT OF ATROPHIC ACNE SCARS USING THE**
MICRONEEDLING WITH DERMAPEN EQUIPMENT IN WOMEN AGED 20 TO 30. Revista científica do
unisalesiano- LINS- SP; ANO 7, N.15, DEZ/2016.

PEREIRA, B.B.; TERRUEL, D.S.; CARRILHO, M.F.B. Treatment of atrophic acne scars using microneedling with dermapen equipment in women aged 20 to 30 years. Revista Científica do Unisalesiano, v.7, n.15, p.1-15, 2016. PEREIRA, B.B.; TERRUEL, D.S.; CARRILHO, M.F.B. Treatment of atrophic acne scars using microneedling with dermapen equipment in women aged 20 to 30 years. **Revista Científica do Unisalesiano,** v.7, n.15, p.1-15, 2016.

PEREIRA, B.B.; TERRUEL, D.S.; CARRILHO, M.EB. Treatment of atrophic acne scars using microneedling with dermapen equipment in women aged 20 to 30 years. Revista Científica do Unisalesiano, v.7, n.15, p.1-15, 2016.

PEREIRA, E.P.L.; CUNHA, M.L.R.S. Evaluation of nasal colonisation by oxacillin-resistant Staphylococcus spp. in nursing students. J Bras Patol Med Lab, v.45, n.5, p.361-369, 2009. Regulatory rewiring confers serotype-specific PRESTES, R.C. et al. Characterisation of collagen fibre, gelatine and hydrolysed collagen. **Revista Brasileira de Produtos Agroindustriais,** v.15, n.4, p.375-382, 2013.

PRETES, R. Collagen and its Derivatives: Characteristics and Applications in Meat Products. UNOPAR **Cient Ciênc Biol Saúde** 2013;15(1):65-74

RIBEIRO, C.M; CARDOSO, T.A.O; **Biosafety:** essential cognitive **approach** to the biologist; Biosafety: an essential cognitive approach for biologists. 2015 Apr-Jun; 9(2) e - ISSN 1981 - 6278

RIBEIRO, Gerusa; PIRES, Denise Elvira Pires de FLOR, Rita de Cássia.
CONCEPTIONS OF BIOSAFETY OF TECHNICAL NURSING TEACHERS IN A SOUTHERN BRAZILIAN STATE. *Trab. educ. saúde.*
2015, vol.13, n.3, pp.721-737. ISSN 1678-1007.

RIBEIRO[1] , G. PIRES[2] , D. E. P. SCHERER[3] , M. D. A. Praticas de biossegurança no ensino técnico de enfermagem; **Biosecurity practices in technical nursing education**; *Praticas de Bioseguridad em La ensenaza tecnica de enfermeria.* **Trab. Educ. Saúde, Rio de Janeiro,** v. 14 n, 3 P.871- 888, Sep./Dec. 2016.

RODRIGUES. DA. Et al; diseases caused by bacteria.**Edtitoraunifesp.** p. 45-58, ISBN 978-85-61,673-68-0, 2010.

ROSA, J.M.; TOKARS, E. The importance of knowing the healing phases for selecting the postoperative aesthetic procedure. 2017

ROSA, R.T.; GONÇALVES, R.B.; ROSA, E.A.R. Transmissibility of streptococcariogens: a conceptual update. Revista Clínica e Pesquisa Odontológica, v.1, n.4, 2005.

Rubin, F.H.; Cerbaro, K.; Naumann, V.; Brunelli, A.V.; Coser, J. **Microbiological evaluation of the hands, utensils, and surfaces of food handlers at the Cruz Alta food bank.** In: Proceedings of the 17th Seminar Interinstitutional Teaching, Research and Extension Exhibition, 15th Scientific Initiation Exhibition and 10th Extension Exhibition; 2012 Nov 6-8; Cruz Alta, Bahia. Cruz Alta: Unicruz; 2012. SANTANA, C. N. L. L.; PEREIRA, D. N.; VASCONCELLOS, J. B.; LACERDA, V. C.; VASCONCELOS, B. N. Microneedling in the treatment of atrophic acne scars: case series. **Surg Cosmet Dermatol**, v. 8, n. 4 (suppl. 1), p. 63-65, 2016.

SANTANA, C.N.L.L.; PEREIRA, D.D.N.; DE VASCONCELLOS, J.N.; LACERDA, V.D.C.; VASCONCELOS, B.N. Microneedling in the treatment of atrophic acne scars: case series. **Surgical & Cosmetic Dermatology**, v. 8, n. 4, 2016. SANTANA, E.H.W. et al. Staphylococci in Food. Arq. Inst. Biol., v.77, n.3, p.545-554, 2010. SANTOS, V.P. Estreptococcias - Streptococcalinfections. Jornal de Pediatria, v.75, n.1, p.103-114, 1999.

SERRANO, G. et al. Microneedling dilates the follicular infundibulum and increases transfollicular absorption of liposomal sepia melanin. **Clinical, Cosmetic and Investigational Dermatology**, v.8, p.313-318, 2015.

SHARMA, O. et al. NAD+-Glycohydrolase Promotes Intracellular Survival of Group A Streptococcus. Journal Plos Pathogens, v.12, n.3, 2016.

SINGH, A.; YADAV, S. Microneedling: Advances and widening horizons. **Indian Dermatology Online Journal**, v. 7, n. 4, p. 244-254, 2016.

SINGH, Aashim; YADAV, Savita. Microneedling: Advancesandwideninghorizons. Indiandermatology online journal, v. 7, n. 4, p. 244, 2016.

Sousa, Álvaro Francisco Lopes de, et al. **"Nursing social representations on biosafety: occupational health and preventive care."** Revista Brasileira de Enfermagem 69.5 (2016): 864-871.

SOUZA, C.S.et al; Soft tissue infections Erysipelas. Cellulitis. Toxin-mediated infectious syndromes. **Symposium: Infectious Urgencies and Emergencies,** v. 36, p.351-356, 2003

STALEY, J. T. & GOSINK. J.**JPoles apart:** biodiversity and biogeography of sea ice bacteria. . 1999.

STALEY, J.. **Microbial Diversity and the Biosphere.** http://www.bdt.org.br/oea/sib/staley. 1998.

STELLA, M.G.; OLIVEIRA, S.P.; Microneedling: percutaneous collagen induction therapy.

Streptoc TANAKA, I.I; IWAMOTO, A.H.; PERSON, O.C.

Acute tonsillitis caused by Streptococcus pyogenes.O Mundo da Saúde, v.33, n.1, p.114-117, 2009.

TONOLLI, V.M.; OCANHA, J.P.; STOLF, H.O. Disseminated bullous impetigo. **Revista Diagnóstico e Tatamento**, v.19, n.3, p.125-128, 2014.

TRABULSI. L.R; ALTERTHUM, F.; **Microbiology.** 5ª edition. São Paulo: Atheneu Publishing House, 2008.

TRINDADE, L.; SANTOS, L.T.R.; SOUZA, A.B.; Analysing the effectiveness of microneedling for acne scars. 2017.

VOMERO, A. et al.Invasive diseases caused by Streptococcuspyogenes 2005-2013. Hospital Pediátrico del Centro Hospitalario Pereira Rossell, Uruguay. Rev. chil. infectol. , v.31, n.6, 2014.

WAJIMA, T. et al. Molecular Characterisation of Invasive Streptococcus dysgalactiae subsp. equisimilis, Japan.Centers for Disease Control and Prevention, v.22, n.2, 2016. WALKER, M.J. et al. Disease Manifestations and Pathogenic Mechanisms of Group A **Streptococcus. Clinical Microbiology Reviews**, v.27, n.2, p.264-301, 2014.

WANG, Y. et al. A precision microbiome approach using sucrose for selective augmentation of **Staphylococcus epidermidis** fermentation against propionibacterium acnes. **International journal of, Molecular Sciences**, v.17, n.11, 2016.

WEBER.C.S; JOAO.F.S.B; LÚCIA. D. M. Cutaneous botryomycosis - case report. **In. Bras. Dermatol.** V. 84, n. 4, p.396-9, 2009.

WINN, W.C, JR. et al. **Microbiological Diagnosis: text and colour atlas.**6ª edition.Rio de Janeiro: Guanabara KooganLtda, 2008

WINN, W.C, JR. et al. **Microbiological Diagnosis: text and colour atlas.** 6ª edition. Rio de Janeiro: Guanabara Koogan Ltda, 2008.

ZANATTA FB, ROSING CK. Chlorhexidine: action's mechanisms and recent evidences of it's efficacy over supragingival biofilm context. **Sci - A.** 2007;1(2):35-43. ZEUGOLIS0, D.I. ; RAGHUNATH , M. Collagen: Materials Analysis and Implant Uses. In: P. Ducheyne, K. Healy, D. Hutmacher, D. Grainger, C. Kirkpatrick (Eds.). **Comprehensive Biomaterials**, 2011. Ed. Elsevier: 261- 278.

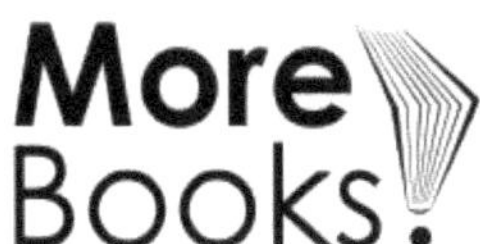

More
Books!

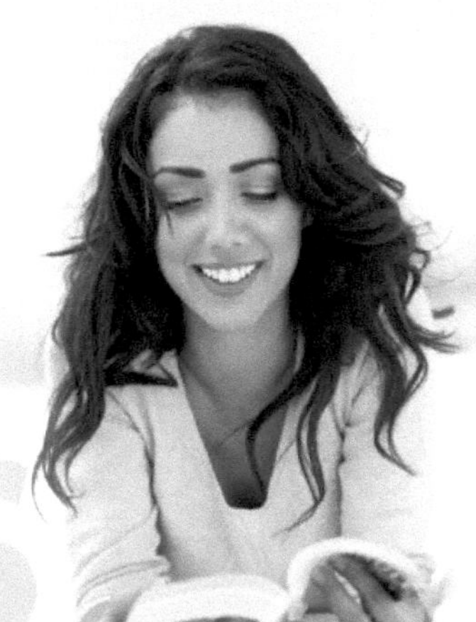

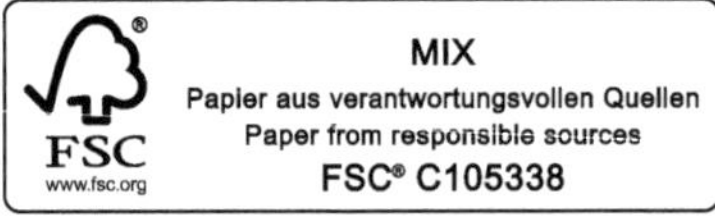

Printed by Books on Demand GmbH, Norderstedt / Germany